When One Door Closes

A Teen's Inspiring Journey and Living Legacy

When One Door Closes

A Teen's Inspiring Journey and Living Legacy

Susie and Bill Graham
with
H. Thomas Saylor

∴ Three Dot L.L.C.
Northville, Michigan

Publisher's Cataloging-in-Publication

Graham, Susie.
    When one door closes : a teen's inspiring journey and
living legacy / by Susie and Bill Graham ; with H.
Thomas Saylor. -- 1st ed.
    p. cm.
    Includes bibliographical references.
    LCCN 2008900651
    ISBN-13: 978-0-9762012-1-2
    ISBN-10: 0-9762012-1-6

    1. Graham, Alexandra--Anecdotes. 2. Terminally ill--
Anecdotes. 3. Bones--Cancer--Patients--Anecdotes.
4. Teenagers--Death--Anecdotes. I. Graham, Bill, 1944-
II. Saylor, H. Thomas. III. Title. IV. Title: Teen's
inspiring journey and living legacy.

    R726.8.G73 2008   362.1'092
                        QBI08-600088

First Edition: August 2008

Book design by Brian Townsend | Select photos courtesy Naturally Photography by Monni

Permissions and Sources

The authors would like to acknowledge the following publishers and individuals for permission to reprint the following material on the pages as noted in order of appearance. (Note: Quotations penned anonymously or in the public domain are not included in this listing. Sources of excerpts and quotations which fall within the realm of fair use are included where possible in appreciation for and to give credit to the fine authors and publishers they represent. Use of such material does not in any way constitute or is it to be construed as an endorsement or recommendation by those authors or publishers.)

Quote page 13: "...the paradox of...is all about" from *Wisdom of the Ages: A Modern Master Brings Eternal Truths to Life* by **Wayne W. Dyer**, Copyright © 1998 by Dr. Wayne W. Dyer. Reprinted by permission of HarperCollins Publishers.

This book is dedicated to:

Make-A-Wish Foundation and its staff, volunteers, donors and supporters who bring hope, strength and joy to the human experience by granting the wishes of children with life-threatening medical conditions,

and to

American Cancer Society and its staff, volunteers, donors and supporters who are dedicated to eliminating cancer as a major health problem by preventing cancer, saving lives and diminishing suffering from cancer through research, education, advocacy and service.

Table of Contents

IV. *The Legacy*

V. *The Challenge*

Acknowledgements

Susan and Bill Graham

We would like to acknowledge the love and support shown by our family and friends both throughout Alex's lifetime and today as we share her story through our individual and collective accounts. Among our family and friends we include and embrace all the caregivers; clergy; physicians and medical personnel; volunteers; and well wishers, who encouraged, counseled and sustained us. For his belief in the value of this project and for his creative and editorial contributions, we wish to thank H. Thomas Saylor.

We also wish to extend a special note of appreciation to all the members, employees, volunteers and supporters of the following:

Adat Shalom Synagogue
American Cancer Society
BERLINE
Caribou Coffee
Detroit Free Press
FOURSIGHT Creative Group, Inc.
Heritage Newspapers
Hillel Day School of Metropolitan Detroit
Israel Cancer Association of Michigan
Joe Dumars Charitable Foundation
Make-A-Wish Foundation of America
Make-A-Wish Foundation of Michigan
Malloy Incorporated
Memorial Sloan-Kettering Cancer Center
News/Talk 760 WJR
Northwest Airlines
Ronald McDonald House Charities
Rose Cancer Center of William Beaumont Hospital
Team Alex
The Detroit News
The Detroit Jewish News
The Oakland Press

The Observer & Eccentric Newspapers
WDIV LOCAL 4
West Bloomfield High School
Wheels for the World
William Beaumont Hospital
WJBK FOX 2
WKQI 95.5
WTVS Detroit Public Television
WWJ Newsradio 950
WXYZ Channel 7

To Bette Midler and the Atlantic Recording Corporation for graciously sharing her rendition of the song, "Wind Beneath My Wings," so that Alex's wish could come true; and to Ed Robertson of the Barenaked Ladies, whose personal time and attention eased the pain and brought a smile to the face of a young patient with cancer, we offer our heartfelt respect and eternal gratitude.

Mostly we are thankful to our sons David and Robbie for their patience, understanding and steadfast love and to our daughter, Alex, for showing all of us that when faced with the worst of adversities, we can still find the courage to go on and the will to open doors for ourselves and for others.

In love and gratitude,

Susie and Bill Graham

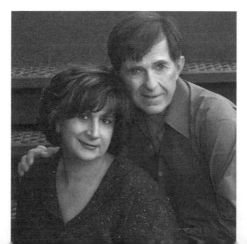

When One Door Closes

A Teen's Inspiring Journey and Living Legacy

Introduction

H. T. Saylor

Life's a bitch and then you die. That's what the bumper sticker read on the SUV in front of me as I inched my car through traffic. I happen not to be a fan of any kind of bumper sticker. Maybe because of my career in the auto industry, I hate to see adhesive-backed paper slapped on expensive clear-coated sheet metal. That said, I admit some of the stickers are exceptionally clever. Many even carry a sincere, well-intentioned message, but the expression "life's a bitch" always makes me wonder. Is it merely a way to vent about the frustrations of the day, or is it something more? Do more of us feel like victims living lives that don't matter?

On that cold February day I found myself much less judgmental of bumper stickers and more sympathetic with the owner of the SUV. My day wasn't going particularly well, and life in general wasn't progressing according to plan. I had taken an early retirement from a Fortune 500 company with hopes of embarking on a less stressful and more fulfilling phase of life. Instead, the Michigan economy turned south, employment opportunities in my field were scarce, and it became obvious that I appeared older in the eyes of potential employers than I perceived myself to be.

Going from a private office on the executive floor to selling my services door to door was a bigger leap than I had anticipated. Freelance work was spotty, and without full-time employment I had more time on my hands than anticipated. The good news was

3

that my flexible schedule allowed me to tackle a couple of writing projects on my personal "to do" list. As I drove down the highway I spotted a strip mall where I could take a break from rush hour and grab a hot cup of coffee. I pulled into the parking lot and noticed a card and gift shop among the storefronts. As long as I was there, I decided to stop in and try to sell a few copies of my work.

The sign over the shop read "Greetings From." Once inside I made my way over to the register, where I was given a warm greeting by a woman behind the counter. I told her that I had a book they might want to add to their gift selection. She said it would be a moment while she went to get the owner. While I waited, I looked around and was encouraged to see the shop also offered a small collection of books.

From the back of the store walked a smartly dressed, dark-haired woman wearing distinctive black-framed glasses. She smiled as she extended her hand to shake mine and said, "Hello. I'm Susan Graham, the owner. Everyone calls me Susie. I understand that you are an author?" I thanked her for her time and handed her a copy of my book for her review. As she paged through the sample, I shared a little about my background in corporate communications and my new career as an independent consultant and writer. She listened politely and offered to take five copies of the book. Mission accomplished.

I began gathering my things to leave and Susie said, "My husband and I have a book we want to write, but we just don't know where to start or how to get it done." I responded, "You do? Well, you should write it. With today's technology the barriers to getting published are not the roadblocks they once were. You know what they say? Everybody has at least one book inside them." Privately I was thinking about the rest of that expression as it was related to me. "And that's where most books by nonprofessionals should stay." I went on, "I really appreciate you displaying my book in your store. I'd be happy to share my experiences and publishing contacts with you when you are ready to make your book happen. What's it going to be about?"

"It's about our daughter, Alex, and her battle with cancer, but it's more than that. It's about the power of a wish and how it changed lives. Our Alex was only 17 when she died, but her message reached people around the world and is still making a difference today. I know her story can encourage and inspire others, especially those facing adversity in their lives."

I felt a surge of guilt after wallowing in my personal situation. What seemed important an hour before paled miserably in comparison to the loss of a child. I offered, "If you want to write this book, maybe I can be of some help. Would you like to talk about that possibility?"

Two weeks later, I met Susie for coffee at a nearby Caribou coffee shop. While I purchased my morning cup of dark roast, Susie found a table where we could sit and talk about her book. As I took my seat she wasted no time in launching into a detailed account of Alex's battle with cancer. As Susie told the story I was moved not only by what I heard but by the emotion and sense of urgency in her voice. I suggested we meet again along with her husband, Bill, to discuss ways they could move their project forward. At the next meeting the three of us talked further and agreed the story they wanted to tell was not only about Alex, but the people she knew and loved. It was about how a life-threatening illness impacts both the individual and that person's family and friends. It was about how the choices we make today can influence the present and the future.

Doors of opportunity and adversity force us to make life-altering decisions. The way in which we respond reflects our character and may one day define our legacy. How would you respond if suddenly you were diagnosed with a life-threatening disease? What if it was someone you loved or a close member of your community? In the pages that follow, guided by excerpts from Alex Graham's journal and commentary by her parents, Susie and Bill, you will be uplifted by a story of courage, determination, love and a wish come true. Listen and learn from the many voices in Alex's life as they share their perspective on what transpired and their personal thoughts on living a life that matters. As you read *When One Door Closes*, gain strength and direction from inspirational quotes, and discover ways you, too, can open doors in your life and in the lives of others.

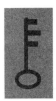

When one door closes, another opens; but we often look so long and so regretfully upon the closed door that we do not see the one which has opened for us.

Alexander Graham Bell
Scientist, inventor and innovator

The Diagnosis

Then Dr. Irwin came into the room and said,
"Well, I've looked at your X-rays, and
I'm 99 percent sure that it's malignant."
I was like, "What?"
Alex asks, "What does malignant mean?"

SUSIE GRAHAM

When One Door Closes

Knock Knock

H. T. Saylor

Remember when you were a child and the doorbell rang? "Mommy! Mommy! Someone is here!" Maybe it's some kind of special surprise, or maybe it's grandma and grandpa coming over to visit and play games. When it was grandma and grandpa, life was good, but sometimes the excitement was quickly followed by disappointment. To this day I can remember standing by my mother's side anticipating the best as she opened the door only to hear the words, "Fuller Brush man. I'll only take a few moments of your time." Those words put a quick damper on my expectations. It was not the guest I wanted, and I knew the next hour would be spent sitting next to my mom listening to a conversation about scrubbing brushes and cleaning solutions.

Then there is the ever-popular "knock-knock" joke, a time-honored format of the pun in which the protagonist says, "Knock, knock!" The antagonist or recipient of the wit answers, "Who's there?" The punster responds with something like, "Doris." The recipient questions, "Doris who?" The punster delivers the punch line, "Doris open and I'm coming in."

In the 1970s the cast members of the late-night comedy television series *Saturday Night Live* took "knock-knock" to a whole new level. While not based on the pun, the arrival of the unexpected knock on the door by the protagonist begs the antagonist to open and let him enter. The skit was called "Land Shark." There would be a knock at the door, and when the homeowner asked "who's there?" a voice would respond, pretending to be everything from a repairman to a candygram delivery. The unsuspecting homeowner, sometimes played by

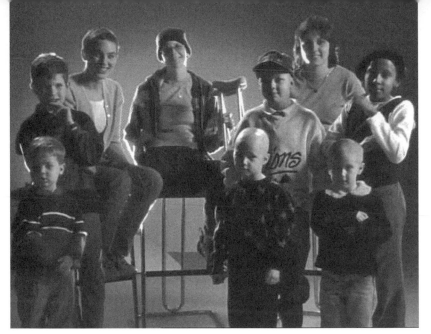

Alex's and friends film her wish for you, "Try a smile."

comedienne and actress, Gilda Radner, would eventually open the door only to be greeted and devoured by a huge "land shark," underscored by the theme from the movie Jaws.

In January of 1999, a group of nine children and teens started making unexpected visits to households throughout America. They weren't there to tell a joke or make a pun, and they weren't there pretending to be someone or something that they weren't. They were knocking at doors fulfilling a wish of their leader, Alex Graham. They were there to help Alex share a message of love, hope and compassion. They were nine beautiful children, each fighting some form of cancer. They were reaching out through Alex's television message, asking for our attention and, not only a change of heart, but a change of mind.

About one year later, they knocked at the door of a young college student in Vermont. When he turned on his television, there they were, sharing this message.

> *Alex and her friends have something to say to you.*
> *Please listen.*

It's not our fault we got sick,
so please don't stare at us because we might look
    a little different.
We're just kids like you.

Sometimes cancer messes up my voice, but I still have
    something to say.
We've already had too many shots, too many
    transfusions and too many chemos.
Too many pokes.

We've had enough hurt in our lives already.
So next time you see a kid with cancer or even
    someone who looks a little different,
try a smile.
We could use it.

This was Alex's Make-A-Wish. We hope you paid
attention.

This is how the young man responded to Alex's message.

To: wishmich@wishmich.org
Date: Thursday, January 13, 2000

Hello,

My name is Greg. I am a student at the University of
Vermont. Today, my friend and I were at her
apartment in Burlington, Vermont, watching one of
our favorite programs on The Learning Channel when
a commercial came on that caught our attention. It was
a commercial about children with cancer. The
commercial was comprised of a group of children
suffering from cancer telling the viewing audience that
they are no different from any other children aside
from their disease. The two of us had never thought
otherwise, but the commercial touched us.

Whereas the stereotypical commercial about disease might showcase the actual suffering and pain of the victims, this commercial took a positive, optimistic approach to the issue. Nothing touched us more than the very last image. After it was made clear that it was a commercial for or from the Make-A-Wish Foundation, there were words on the screen that said, "This was Alex's wish. We hope you paid attention."

Tears of... something rushed to my eyes. I was blown away that this young woman's wish had been such a selfless act; that more than anything in the world that she could have wished for, she chose only to send a wonderful, meaningful, touching message to the world, to contribute to making the world a better place for us to live in. I turned around and saw that my friend's eyes were also watery. I knew right away that I had to tell someone how much we were moved by this wish. That is why I am writing.

I am not personally in need of any wish, but I do have a wish to ask for and hope that it would be possible for you to grant. I would really like Alex to know how far her wish has reached. I guess I would like to say to her, "Alex, we were paying attention. Thank you and keep up the wonderful work."

Take care,

Greg

When Greg turned on the television that day he did not anticipate Alex and her friends knocking at his door. He did not expect to be emotionally moved by a message from someone he did not know. He was unaware of the courageous battle Alex Graham had fought with cancer, and he knew nothing of her fate. What he did know was that Alex's wish was alive, meaningful and making a difference.

We never know when there will be an unexpected knock at our door. Sometimes we can choose not to answer. Sometimes, like in the pun shared earlier, the visitor declares, "Doris open and I'm coming in." Ironically, that is what happened to comedienne Gilda Radner when in 1986 she was diagnosed with ovarian cancer. Unlike the "Land Shark" skit, this time a real predator was at her door. That is exactly what Alex Graham faced in 1997 when she was diagnosed with a cancerous tumor. Without permission and undetected, cancer invaded her young body and challenged Alex to the ultimate battle of survival.

Illness and tragedy can arrive in our lives at any time and often does so when least expected. The way in which we respond to our circumstance can change our lives and our legacy forever. When illness and tragedy enter our household it not only impacts an individual but one's entire family and circle of friends. Such was the case with Alex Graham, her family and her community. To fully appreciate her story and its lasting influence we need to go back to the beginning when her parents, Susie and Bill first met.

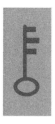

...the paradox of the statement, "doomed to make choices," is evident at all times. That is, we are in control, and we are not in control, all at the same time, and learning to live with this enigma is a big part of what knowing God is all about.

Wayne W. Dyer, Ph.D.
Author, *Wisdom of the Ages*

When Susie Met Billy

Susie Graham

My dreams were like any young girl's dreams. I was born and raised in the Detroit area, as were my parents and grandparents. I had visions of a career in social work and eventually having a husband and family. When it came time for me to go to college, I enrolled at Eastern Michigan University. That's where this big-city girl met and fell in love with a small-town boy named William. William, or Billy, as his family called him, was from a nearby rural community where the gas station was "the" gas station and the drug store was "the" drug store. While our backgrounds and many of our opinions differed, we both came from hard-working, close-knit, supportive families. We shared core values, and it wasn't long before we grew to share a love that could not be denied. Two years after we met, Billy and I were wed. I was 20 years old, and Billy was 23.

About three years later we decided to start a family. A year passed, and I still wasn't pregnant. We finally consulted a doctor and found out that the chances of having a child were slim. We decided to adopt, and before long our first son, David came to us when he was two months old. We were in our twelfth year of marriage when we were surprised and delighted to learn I was pregnant with our second son, Robert. He and David are five and a half years apart.

At the age of three David was diagnosed with hyperactivity and attention deficit disorder. He had a lot of trouble in his nursery school settings, and as the years went by, the whole school experience became a nightmare for him. We took him to counseling, and he was placed on Ritalin. Generally he did pretty well with the academics, and together we did well in our family setting. It was something else in the mix—other kids, other people, other distractions that exacerbated the hyperactivity.

David was very devoted to the family, and we were crazy about him, but as far as school and life outside the family unit, David was going right down the tubes. We enrolled him at Eton Academy which is a school for children with learning disabilities. He didn't like Eton at all. He made sure he got into enough mischief so they would not want him back. By the time he got to high school, we decided something had to be done. He got in a bit of trouble outside of school, and, after consulting with a specialist, we sent him to a school called Grove in Madison, Connecticut. David took part in the decision too. He knew he needed help that he couldn't get at home. Grove specialized in working with kids who had high IQs and emotional problems. There they were able to catch things as they happened and work with David on an individual basis.

So while we are trying to help David, along came our other son Robbie. He was a great kid. He was cute and charming, and everybody loved him. He went to Hillel, a Jewish elementary day school not far from our home. Between his personality and the supportive environment at the school, Robbie made his way, but it wasn't long before problems began to surface. It turned out that like his older brother, he was also learning-disabled. He was diagnosed with dysgraphia, a medical condition that limits an individual's ability to express thoughts in writing and write legibly. Robbie was experiencing increased difficulty with his classes, and I found myself thinking, "Oh my God! We just went through all this with David. What else is in store for us?"

When Robbie finished Hillel, he wanted to go to Roeper High School, but because of his learning disability, his academic qualifications did not meet enrollment guidelines. Robbie, just an eighth grader, took it upon himself to compose a letter. In the letter he wrote, "I need to get into your school. I think I can do well. I need to get into your school or I'll kill myself." I told him, "You don't need the 'I'll kill myself' thing." A week or two later a Roeper representative called and said, "We often get letters from parents requesting admission for their child, but this is the first time we received such a letter written by the student." In great part because of his letter, Roeper asked Robbie to come in for an interview, and eventually accepted him as a student.

A few months into the fall semester, Robbie started to have trouble. Because of the dysgraphia, his Spanish teacher could not read our son's writing. Robbie was forced to take his exams on a computer. In math, he couldn't write the problems either. According to his algebra teacher, Robbie could actually come close to solving the problems in his head, but couldn't express them legibly and accurately on paper. Like David, Robbie was bright, but had a hard time keeping up because of a learning disability. Robbie figured he was bright too—so bright, that he wanted to quit school.

Both of our boys were struggling. Like any parent, it was heartbreaking to watch them go through difficult times, so Billy and I found ourselves struggling right along with them. It seemed like we were constantly asking, "What's the best thing we can do for our sons now?"

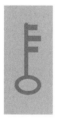

We're all gathered at a doorway today. It's the end of something and the beginning of something else.

Alan Alda
Author, *Things I Overheard While Talking to Myself*

When One Door Closes

Along Came Alex
Susie

Alex was a typical adolescent. She was great to her friends yet all about herself. She was sometimes moody but usually funny. In fact, she loved to be the clown. I guess you'd say she was a pretty normal teenager.

Eighth Grade Teacher

Eleven months after Robbie was born, I was pregnant again. I was trying not to think, "Oh, it would be really nice to have a girl." But when they said it was a girl, I remember being so excited! She was so small and precious. The first thing I did when I was able to get up and around was to go buy Alex a pink dress.

I remember people would say, "Oh, girls—you know they are really tough to raise." I thought, "How tough can it be? My husband, Billy, is a workaholic, my oldest son is hyperactive with attention deficit disorder, and Robbie has dysgraphia. We have somehow managed to deal effectively with those conditions, so raising a daughter can't possibly be more challenging. As it turned out, Alex was a very, very easy child to raise. She even toilet trained herself. Amazingly, she was never sick. She was never, ever sick.

Like Robbie, Alex went to the Hillel Day School. At first I wasn't sure I wanted them to go there, but at the first orientation I met the headmaster who was the rabbi there. He said, "I want to tell you about one of the most important reasons for coming to Hillel. When one of the children has a birthday party, you invite all the kids in the class to the birthday party. In other words, everyone is fully included here." That's when I said, "This is the school for our children." I felt Hillel was unique too, because they not only offered the academics, and the biblical lessons, but they really stressed to the kids how important it was to teach and share with others.

She loved going to school there; partly because she loved Judaism and partly because she was very social. Classes, on the other hand, weren't always easy for her. She had a bit of a reading comprehension difficulty, so she wasn't an "A" student. A lot of her friends were, and because she always wanted to do her best, she wasn't shy about asking for help. "Hey, I'm having trouble with this. Can you help me? Can you come and study with me because I am really having trouble with that?" She wasn't afraid to speak up either. One time when one of the teachers was soundly scolding one of the boys in her class, Alex just got up and said, "There's no reason for you to talk to him that way." Alex quickly found herself outside of the classroom being talked to by the teacher. Years later, the teacher admitted, "I didn't appreciate the disruption she caused in the classroom, but privately I really admired her for that."

Alex was indeed a teacher and an intermediary. If Billy and I were having an argument, she would say, "Mom, just go tell dad you love him." She was also very protective of her brother, David. While seven and a half years younger than he, she was always saying, "We have to be more patient with David. We have to be more patient." She would do that with friends too. If a couple of her friends were angry with each other, Alex would walk a fine line between the two points of view. Somehow she would find a way to mediate and keep both friends in the process.

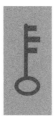

Normal day, let me be aware of the treasure you are. Let me learn from you, love you, bless you before you depart.

Mary Jean Iron
Poet

The Brothers

David and Robbie Graham

Watching Robbie and Alex was a challenge. Alex knew just how to antagonize Robbie and he was always quick to respond. Not everyone saw that Alex was pushing his buttons, but she was a master at it.

Cousin and Babysitter, Bethany

What was it like growing up in the Graham household? Let's see. Being the oldest of three, I guess I'd characterize it as unorganized and a bit insane. My mom would try to keep it together, but my dad would make it insane. He worked a lot too, so he wasn't home much of the time. That was probably a good thing. Of course, my brother Robbie and I didn't help matters at all. My room was always a mess, his room was always a mess, and we did our part to keep the whole house a mess.

The two of us fought constantly as brothers often do. Robbie was the event and project creator. He always seemed to have something going on around the house like a carnival. My friends and I would try to disrupt it. Robbie would call me a name. I'd call him a name. He'd hit me. I'd hit him back, and he'd start crying. I'd lock myself in my room, and the next day we would do it all over again.

I was seven and a half years older than my sister Alex, so we really didn't hang out much. You know how girls don't like big brothers interfering with their fun and games. Don't get me wrong. We loved each other, but for me it was another opportunity to keep things interesting. Alex's friends would come over, and I'd find ways to tease them and embarrass her. At that stage she was a bit of a whiner, so it made teasing all that more rewarding.

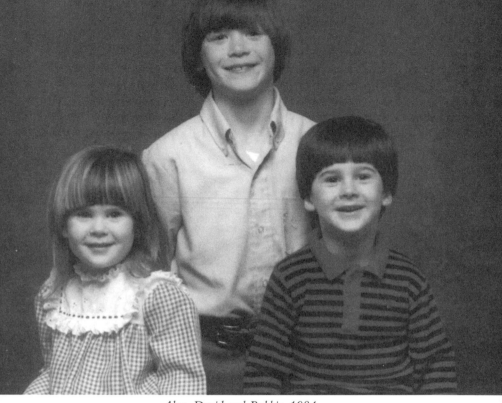

Alex, David and Robbie, 1984

★ ★ ★ ★ ★

David's right. I was the doer, the planner, the entrepreneur. I remember one time I really wanted this remote-control car. I had about $100 saved up but was still short of my goal. Well, my room was bigger than Alex's. I convinced her she really wanted a bigger room then sold it to her to get the rest of the funds I needed. My parents were like, "What the heck are you doing?"

Then there was the time when they were building the back half of our subdivision. To me it was an opportunity ripe for the picking. I took our picnic table, turned it upside down, and put caster wheels on it. Then I loaded it up with chips, candy and a cooler filled with pop. I pushed it through the construction site and took in a whopping $35 to $40 a day.

When I wasn't doing that, I was mowing lawns. I mean, how many kids do you know who get a riding lawnmower for

When One Door Closes

their bar mitzvah? By the time I was 16 years old I was renting and running a Bobcat for my own landscape company. Finally, things really started getting out of hand when I drove a dump truck to school. By then, I didn't see a need for school. I mean, my classmates are talking about the TV program *90210*, and I was out signing contracts with a chain of auto service stations to landscape, mow and plow nine of their properties.

Next thing you know, I dropped out of high school. My parents said, "If you're not going to school then it's time you started paying rent or else get your own apartment." "Or else" sounded good to me. I moved out.

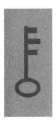

Brothers and sisters help each other along, first up backyard hills, and later up lifelong climbs.

William Bennett
American author and politician

Alex the Athlete

Bill Graham

My daughter was very much an individualist. She did her own thing and was not concerned about what other people thought.

Susie

I enjoy sports, and Alex did too. She and I had a close father-daughter relationship and athletics was one of the interests we shared. Alex loved to play and compete, and I loved watching and being a proud parent.

One time she was participating in the Maccabi Games. Maccabi USA/Sports for Israel is a volunteer organization that seeks to enrich the lives of Jewish youth through sports competition much like the Catholic Youth Organization. This particular year the games were in Los Angeles. Susie and I were among the parents there watching, and Alex won a gold medal in the 13- and 14-year-old girls' 3000 meter run. She was then scheduled to be in a relay event and to everyone's surprise asked the coach if she could skip it. The coach was puzzled and said to her, "Alex, you are one of our best runners. Why in the world would you want to skip an event?" Alex replied, "Because I want my friend to run with my team instead, so she can win a medal too." Coach thought for a minute and replied, "Alex, your friend has to win her own medal, and you're running for our fastest team." As it turned out, several runners including Alex tripped in the race. Her friend's relay team ended up placing and winning a medal. This wish for Alex came true. Her friend experienced the joy of winning and was awarded the medal that Alex wanted her to have.

Growing up, Alex played other sports too. She wasn't the best baseball player, but on or off the field, she was rooting for her team. She was always there trying her hardest…giving her best. In high school she tried out for softball but didn't make the squad. I was disappointed for her, but there was always running. In that sport she was a natural with loads of potential. She ran so effortlessly that her track coach and I really wanted to see what she could do in cross country. Instead, one day she said, "Dad, I like to run, but I've decided to work at the children's daycare center."

So much for cross country, but Alex knew what she wanted. She went to work part-time for a home-based daycare center. There she demonstrated another kind of natural talent: the ability to work with kids. Privately the owner of the daycare shared with Susie and me what an inspiration Alex was to her and how gifted Alex was at working with the children.

I wanted Alex to run cross country. She wanted to work in a daycare center. It's a life lesson I learned. You can't live your child's life for them, and sometimes you are the one who learns the most from the choices they make.

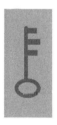

Children need parents who will let them grow up to be themselves, but parents often have personal agendas they try to impose on their children.

Harold S. Kushner
Author, How Good Do We Have To Be?

My Knee Is Bothering Me

Susie

Alex's favorite outfits were jeans, T-shirt, a zippered top and tennis shoes. She never got into name-brand clothes and usually kept things simple. She liked having her own identity and was sometimes upset when she felt others were copying her look.

Susie

By 1997 our three children were more or less independent, but Alex and I remained particularly close. Yes, we were mother and daughter, but we were also really good friends. It was also a time when I was feeling a bit more freedom as an individual. With the children older, I decided I wanted to do something on my own. I planned to open a card, gift and stationery shop, and that June I signed a lease for retail space in a nearby strip mall.

As far as my children's health, if they said they were not feeling well I wouldn't blow them off. I wasn't overly concerned about every little ache and pain, but I listened and observed. One time a doctor said to me, "The best barometer you have on how your child is doing is you. Don't be afraid to call and say, "I don't know what's wrong but my child isn't acting right." I always felt in tune with what was going on with them. That's how I felt in September of 1997.

It was a fairly ordinary September day. Alex had gone to the mall with her friends, and when she came back she said, "You know, mom, I think I may have twisted my knee or something, because it is really bothering me." I'm like, "Okay. Well, let's keep an eye on it for a couple of days and see what happens. If it doesn't get any better, we'll go get an X-ray." I mean, Alex was just never sick, so if she's complaining, I'm listening.

It kept bothering her, so one night we ended up taking her to the emergency room at a local hospital. They did an X-ray on her knee but couldn't find anything. They said, "Here, we'll give you an Ace bandage. Wrap it and see what happens. If it doesn't improve in a week, make an appointment to see your family pediatrician."

A week went by and Alex was still complaining. It was the end of the month, and I said, "You know what? We're going to go to an orthopedic specialist and have him take a look." So I took her to who was supposed to be one of the best doctors in the area. He took another X-ray, and he didn't see anything either. He asked Alex, "Did you ever have an injury to your knee?" Alex answered, "As a matter of fact I did. When I was 14 I was skiing and had a little run in with a tree." He said, "Well, it's possible that there is a little bone chip or something behind your kneecap that's aggravating the joint. Why don't we first try physical therapy? The clinic is right here in the building. Let's see if that remedies the situation. We'll give therapy three weeks and see what happens. If that doesn't help, we'll do laparoscopic surgery to see exactly what's going on behind the kneecap."

For three weeks Alex tried the physical therapy, but there was no sign of improvement. So, in mid October, she had laparoscopic surgery. When the surgery was over, the surgeon came out of the operating room, and I remember the blank look on his face. He said, "I didn't find anything. You know, I just didn't find anything. I just don't know what it is. Maybe your daughter needs some more physical therapy."

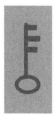

Trust your hunches. They're usually based on facts filed away just below the conscious level.

Joyce Brothers, Ph.D.
Psychologist and columnist

Childhood Friends

Friend Tracie

Journal Entry:

I'm so glad I have family and friends who love me so much.
I never want to lose that feeling.

Alex

Alex and I met in kindergarten. We both went to Hillel Day School, and we lived in the same neighborhood. We were the best of friends throughout elementary and middle school. We spent summer camps together and went to high school together. Because our homes were nearby, we spent a lot of our free time with one family or the other.

A lot of times as you grow up, you grow apart from your early friendships. It didn't happen with us. Sure, we became active in our own interests and with other groups, but we always remained close. We could always go back to each other and pick up right where we left off.

Over the years we spent a lot of time together. We'd do the typical things that kids do; like go to the movies and to the mall. We'd go on vacation with each other's families. Sometimes I would head north with her family to places like Traverse City. Other times she would accompany my family on our vacation trips.

Alex was very outgoing. She was happy-go-lucky. She always seemed to have this positive outlook on life. She had a lot of friends and could always float with ease among the different groups. Alex was a comfortable girl. She let you in. She was one of those people who was well liked by everyone but kind of jokester, too. No matter what you did with Alex, you would end up with this crazy story to tell.

One time we went on a trip with my family to Sugarloaf, a ski resort in northern Michigan. While we were there Alex and I met this crazy little girl. I don't even remember how we met. We didn't even know her name. All we knew was that she was from Sterling Heights, Michigan. So as only Alex could do, she just started calling her Sterling Heights. Alex would go around yelling, "Sterling Heights! Sterling Heights!" I know it's silly, but from that time on, every time we heard anything on the news or whatever that mentioned Sterling Heights, we thought about the girl we met on that ski trip and laughed. Maybe you had to be there, but for a couple of teenage girls, it was the kind of thing that made life fun.

Actually, it was on the trip to Sugarloaf that Alex took her first skiing lessons. Eager to try out her newly acquired skills, Alex struck out on her own. Observers say she was like a maniac going down the hill and ended up crashing into a tree. My mom doesn't ski, so she was at the lodge when she heard the page. The ski patrol had found Alex. When she hit the tree, she injured her knee. Alex took it in stride, but that was the end of skiing for that trip.

About a year later my mom had to have a hysterectomy. At the same time Alex was recovering from her laparoscopic knee surgery. It was odd, because while my mom's surgery was considered major, she kept getting better and better while Alex's knee kept getting worse.

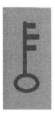

Friends are the sunshine of life.

John Hay
American statesman and author

A Love for Photography and Music

Friend Jessica

Alex didn't hesitate to speak up. Sometimes it was a bit inappropriate. Sometimes it was just her sense of humor. She loved it. I remember the time she told our rabbi that I fell asleep during his sermon.

Bill

Growing up together as childhood friends, it was interesting to watch Alex morph from someone heavy into athletics into a teenager with an artistic focus. Alex did all right in school, but academics weren't her strong suit. While she still liked sports, she loved photography and music even more. After high school, instead of going to one of the many state universities, she talked about enrolling at the Center for Creative Studies in Detroit to study photography. Alex had this unmistakable creative spirit, and photography was an ideal way for her to express her emotions. I think she could see things through the lens the rest of us would overlook, and that's how she was with life. She could see and appreciate what many of us never saw.

As teenagers we were all into one kind of music or another. I liked rap and pop. Alex liked some of that too, but her musical interests were more diverse. I think her parents introduced her to the artists and the music they enjoyed, and because of that Alex gained a broader appreciation than the average teen. Harry Chapin, Carly Simon, and Cat Stevens were among her favorites. She liked Counting Crows, Joni Mitchell, Jackson Browne, Al

Green and Ben Harper. She also liked Peter Paul and Mary, Chava Alberstein and an occasional Otis Redding selection. She liked show tunes and would sometimes break out into a medley from *The Lion King*. She liked Bette Midler, and one of her favorite songs was the Midler version of "Wind Beneath My Wings," released in 1989. I remember too there was one song she really liked by Billy Joel. It was "She's Always a Woman." Alex would say, "I know that song is about me. I love that song." Whenever it came on the radio and we heard it start with the words, "She can kill with her smile, she can wound with her eyes..." the two of us just would crack up. Alex would scream, "It's my song!" It was always good for a laugh, and she was right. I think a good part of that song did describe Alex.

There were serious musical moments too. Alex had this way of being wild and crazy one minute and serious the next. One time we were driving back from the mall, and the song "I'll be Missing You" by P. Diddy and Faith Evans came on. It was a remake of the song originally made popular by the group Police, titled "Every Breath You Take." P. Diddy released his version after the death of rapper Notorious B.I.G. The lyrics say something like, "One day when this life is over I'll see your face..." Alex asked me, "Have you ever thought about your funeral?" I'm thinking, "Wow, where did that come from?" We went on to have this long conversation about life and death. We talked about what our funerals might be like, what would be said and who might be there. It's not the discussion you would expect from two teenage girls, but with Alex, the unexpected was quite typical.

Alex liked what I'd call "feel-good" music, and she was really into laughter and living for the moment. I think that is one of the reasons why she enjoyed the Barenaked Ladies so much. I mean, we all liked BNL, but Alex just loved them. They are a bit quirky, and frankly, Alex was too. *Rolling Stone* magazine once described BNL's humor as, "...a complex wellspring of sources: insecurity, intelligence, neurosis, compassion, alienation, joy, anger and arrested development." There is no doubt the Barenaked Ladies love to laugh and have a good time, and it's evident in their music and their performances. In a way, that was Alex too.

She was this endless source of positive energy. Combined with a sometimes outrageous sense of humor, she had a knack for turning the ordinary into the fun and memorable. But, like her favorite group, she was far more complex than that. Alex not only enjoyed the melody, she contemplated the lyrics. She didn't just snap a photo; she wanted to capture the moment. She didn't just live life, she embraced it.

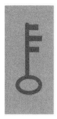

We shun the thought of death as sad, but death will only be sad to those who have not thought of it. It must come sooner or later, and when he who has refused to seek the truth in life will be forced to do so in death.

Francois Fenelon
French Roman Catholic theologian, poet and writer

We May Have a Malignancy

Susie

Journal Entry December 19, 1997:

Alex is in a lot of pain when she walks. She is having trouble sleeping at night. There seems to be swelling above the kneecap.

Susie

Alex's leg continued to hurt so we continued with the therapy. It was the therapist who finally said, "You know, Mrs. Graham, if I were you I would get a second opinion on Alex's knee."

I was like, "Well okay. We need to try something." No one has helped yet and the physical therapy clearly wasn't working. Her leg was all swollen and her knee was more painful than ever. The orthopedic specialist we had been seeing happened to be in the same building as the therapist, so I called him up and said, "Look, it is still hurting her. Your physical therapist is telling us that we need a second opinion. I think you need to see her again."

He took a look at Alex's knee, and you could see him turn pale. It was like a light went on. He clearly knew something. He said, "I want you to go see Dr. Ronald Irwin right now." I asked, "Now?" He said, "Yes, now. There's a mass there."

I wasn't making the connection with what he was saying. A mass? Maybe it's water on the knee or something. He said, "I'm calling Dr. Irwin's office. He'll see you right now. Take this slip. He's waiting for you."

So we went to Dr. Irwin's office and took along the X-rays. Alex and I were physically there, but our minds did not comprehend the gravity of the situation. We were just moving along to the next step in the process as directed. We went in the waiting room, and there the nurse handed us this paper. It read the words, "Specializing in limb salvation." I felt a chill rush over my body. I didn't say anything to Alex. Billy wasn't there, and I was getting really scared.

Then Dr. Irwin came into our room and said, "Well, I've looked at your X-rays, and I'm 99 percent sure that it's malignant." I was like, "What?" Then Alex asked, "What does malignant mean?"

I immediately called Billy. I was feeling hysterical, but I knew that somehow I had to keep it together in front of Alex. "Hi, Billy. We are with Dr. Irwin. You know, Alex needs to have an MRI. We may have a malignancy."

I was devastated, and I don't think Alex had grasped the gravity of what had just transpired.

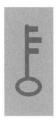

Can you accept the idea that some things happen for no reason, that there is a randomness in the universe?

Harold S. Kushner
Author, *When Bad Things Happen to Good People*

My Leg Has Cancer

Susie

Journal Entry December 22, 1997:

Today was one of the hardest days of my life. I found out I have a cancerous tumor. I'm really scared, but my family and friends are comforting me.

Alex

We were all in shock. Dr. Irwin told us that Alex needed to have an MRI, but we still didn't really know what it all meant. MRIs were not readily available in 1997 and hard to get on short notice, especially in late December. We were fortunate and got one scheduled. By then we were using the term "malignant." Alex knew we were talking about "cancer." Alex knew the whole thing. The situation had taken a dramatic turn. In one day Alex went from a mere sense of uncertainty to someone telling her that she had a malignancy. Now Alex was really scared.

Alex went in for the MRI but had a hard time with the procedure. She always had trouble staying still for long periods of time, and the MRI chamber made her feel claustrophobic. Alex was so upset she couldn't hold still for a successful scan. They had to stop the procedure.

We called Dr. Irwin, because we didn't know what to do. He said, "Well, I can give her something to calm her down to help her get through the MRI." So we tried to get another appointment for the test. They said it would be impossible to get her into the schedule right away. We were panicking. Billy called them in tears. I think that was the only thing that made the difference. They squeezed her back in the appointment schedule. Alex took the Valium to calm down, and this time they were able to successfully complete the test.

The next step in the process was a biopsy. Dr. Irwin deferred a trip to see his ailing father so he could do it himself. The biopsy confirmed what Dr. Irwin expected. It was malignant. Alex indeed had cancer.

Later that day, Alex had a friend over to visit. They were in the basement, and she yelled up the stairway, "Mom..." And I'm like, "Yeah." She goes, "Do I have cancer? You know, don't you, that it's my leg that has cancer? I don't." It turned out to be an expression and a perspective that stuck with all of us.

"I don't have cancer. My leg has cancer."

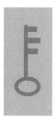

I have no interest in cancer. It may have an interest in me, but I have none in it.

Anonymous cancer patient

Alex just days before the cancer diagnosis.

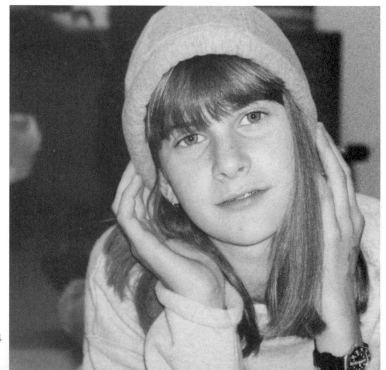

We Need to Sit Down and Talk

Robbie

Journal Entry December 23, 1997:

I had my biopsy. My tumor is called osteogenic sarcoma. I love everyone and it made me feel so good to see who stood by me when I needed them.

Alex

I remember the day. I'm not even sure why I came home. I was immersed in my own life and my business ambitions. Anyway, I came home and my parents are sitting at the table crying. They said, "Robert, we need to sit down and talk."

Now that's a line I had heard a number of times, and it never meant anything good. Growing up, because of all the chaos in the household and all the fighting between us kids, I always had this fear that my parents were going to get divorced. So I came home and they were crying. In my mind I was like, "Oh, they're probably just getting a divorce." With half of my friends having divorced parents, it was almost to be expected. Whatever it was, we would all just have to deal with it.

"Your sister has cancer."

When I heard that, I was thinking, "That isn't good news, but it's not a divorce." I mean, it was 1997. Cancer was curable, or so I thought. It just didn't seem like that big a deal. To me it was like a broken arm. You go, they fix it, you get a cast on it, and before long you're as good as new.

I told my parents, "It will be all right." I was still thinking, "You go to the hospital, they take care of it, and you get up and go on with life."

I was an 18-year-old boy. It was just like, you know, I cared, but I figured everything would be fine.

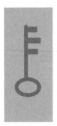

Some children may become very upset when learning about a new cancer diagnosis, while others may act as if nothing is wrong. The goal is to give the child a balanced point of view. The child should realize that cancer is a serious—but not a hopeless—illness.

American Cancer Society
www.cancer.org

You're Going to Beat This!

Friend Jason

Journal Entry December 24, 1997:

Today I had an echocardiogram. That's where they give your heart an ultrasound. Later I'm having a CAT scan.

Alex

My buddy and I were juniors at North Farmington High School. He was always talking about this one particular girl. He said he liked talking to her, and she was really cool. I figured he had a crush on her or something, but he said, "No, she is just fun to be around. I really like talking to her."

This went on for a long time. He was always talking about this Alex girl. So finally I'm like, "Well, maybe you should introduce me to her." He says. "Sure. I'll set it up. The three of us will go hang out at the mall."

So a few days later we are at the mall waiting for Alex to get dropped off. This car pulls up and out steps this good-looking girl. I see she is a bit taller than me, and before you know it she goes, "Hey, you're shorter than me!" I'm thinking that's a pretty out-of-nowhere comment from someone you just met. This girl is really blunt. I think I like that.

The day went great. The three of us walked around the mall for hours. Alex had this off-the-wall sense of humor. We had a lot of laughs just talking, people watching and goofing around. It wasn't too many days after that, and the three of us were hanging out together again. I really liked spending time with her. I thought, "You know, maybe there could be something between us."

So I started calling her now and then. Once in a while she would call me.

I guess I liked her more than she liked me. In time I got the impression that she liked this other guy. She didn't say much to the contrary, and finally I got all mad. I stopped calling and talking to her at all. I figured, "Who needs this. She likes someone else, and there are plenty of other girls out there for me." During the following summer, my buddy and I ran into her at a miniature golf place. She was with a bunch of her friends, and I decided to completely ignore her. She liked someone else, and it made me mad. Apparently I liked her a bit more than I was willing to admit to myself. My buddy still talked about her now and then, but for me, my friendship with her was over before it really got started.

That December, my friends and I were at a youth organization talent show. I spotted Alex in the crowd. I hadn't talked to her in months. I had no plans to change that, but I didn't know my plans were about to change.

After the show my buddy came up to me and said, "Oh, remember Alex? Yesterday they found out she has cancer." I'm like, "No way! Oh, my God. That's horrible." Of course, I knew nothing about cancer at the time. I knew it was a bad thing, but that's about it.

Alex was standing with a bunch of her friends. As I walked closer I could hear them talking about cancer. Alex was filling them in on everything that had happened and the diagnosis. I made my way up to her. She seemed a bit surprised to see me. I said something like, "I'm sorry to hear you're sick. How are you?"

Alex said, "Well, not good."

"If you need anything, call me. I want to get back in touch. I miss talking to you."

The next day I called her. We talked for a little while but not about her illness. We just talked. I called again the next day, and that time we talked about the cancer. I found out she had to go to the hospital for some kind of treatment or test. After the test we talked again. I asked her, "What is this cancer? What's the deal?"

Alex said, "I'm really scared. What if I die from this? I'm really, really scared."

"I promise you, Alex. You are not going to die from cancer."

"No, really. What if this kills me? I'm so scared."

"Alex, I promise you you're going to beat this. Don't worry. You are not going to die. I promise you. You are going to beat this!"

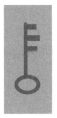

People who are ill are very real. The struggle is their issue. Being involved—seeing, feeling, and caring—is our issue.

Rabbi Alon Tolwin
Director of Aish HaTorah of Metro Detroit

When a Teenager Has Cancer

Jill Elder, American Cancer Society

Journal Entry December, 1997:

My parents have been so strong through all this. I love them.

Alex

I was in college when my brother Jay was diagnosed with cancer. He was 14 years old, and just starting to play football. He was just starting to go out with people who could drive. He was just starting to get into teenage mischief, and Jay was very much a troublemaker.

We think he was probably experiencing some symptoms for a long time that he wasn't articulating. It was actually his football coach that noticed Jay's gait was off. He was missing tackles he would normally make and he was moving and reacting slower. He would choke every time he tried to drink something but never when he ate something. My mom would say, "Slow down! Chew your food!" What Jay didn't share was that he couldn't urinate. Jay's pediatrician who happened to be medical partners with the team doctor ordered an MRI. Nothing prepares you for, "Your son or brother or friend has a brain tumor." It was the last thing we ever expected to hear about a teenage boy in the prime of his life.

Jay was diagnosed in 1995. At that time my first impulse was to go to the library and wipe the dust off the books and figure out what it all meant. Just ten years ago you would come home from the doctor with this big binder. You would start frantically flipping through the pages looking for answers. It was almost archaic. Two years later Alex Graham and her family faced the same cumbersome search for information and answers.

Today there have been great strides in information technology and content and resource information availability. It's one of the reasons why I chose a career with the American Cancer Society and one of the things for which I am most proud. ACS is dedicated to eliminating cancer by prevention and saving lives. We also strive to diminish suffering through research, education, advocacy and service. In 1997 when Alex was diagnosed we didn't have a 24-hour-a-day National Cancer Information Center or an American Cancer Society web site that includes an interactive cancer resource center containing in-depth information on every major cancer type. There wasn't a directory of medical resources with links to other sites organized by cancer type or topic. Neither Alex and her family nor Jay and our family had access to the resources that are available today.

So over time, some things have changed for the better, but then again, when a teenager has cancer, much is the same. Cancer seems to come out of nowhere at a time in their lives when they are just establishing their independence and should have some of the very best days of their lives right within their grasp. They are also at that very "sensitive-about-your-looks" stage of life. Now they are faced with things like losing their hair or extreme weight loss or, in cases where they are put on steroids, ravenous hunger and weight gain. Suddenly their whole world changes and so does that of their parents, their siblings and their friends. Everyone within the family and its circle of relationships is affected. How each reacts and the choices they make can have a profound effect on the situation and on their lives for years to come.

One thing I have noticed about kids with cancer is they suddenly have this unbelievable sense of wisdom. I remember before Jay became ill my mom would say things like, "If something happened to one of my kids, I'd go crazy. They would have to lock me away." Jay remembered that and while going through his treatment he would say to her, "You can't do that, mom. You don't have that option. You've got other things you need to do in life." Teenagers can become so very intuitive and really pay attention to interesting details. In Jay's case it was like he went from a boy to a teen to a man overnight. He guided us through his cancer, and while I never knew Alex personally, I believe that is what she did for her family and friends. I mean, as we get older, we ponder the question, "What will be my legacy?" Then in contrast, you have these teenagers with cancer who would never ask, "What is my legacy?" They just go forward and create it.

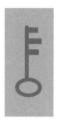

An awareness of one's mortality can lead you to wake up and live an authentic, meaningful life.

Bernie S. Siegel, M.D.
Author, *Love, Medicine & Miracles*

The Journey

Journal Entry:

Today was the best day. All the people I needed
were there for me. I am so lucky to have
so many people near me when I am sad.

ALEX

When It's Your Child's Best Friend

Family Friend Merle

Susie Graham and I met in a "mother-toddler" class. My son is the same age as Alex's brother Robbie and my daughter and Alex were born just five days apart. With the kids' ages in common, Susie and I quickly bonded as friends, and so did our children. It seemed like the kids were together all the time. After the boys started attending different schools, they each went more or less their own way. It was different with my daughter and Alex. They went to different schools after kindergarten, but their relationship was different. They stayed very, very close.

Alex went to Hillel Day School and my daughter went to the public school system. When they had birthdays, they would have their own birthday parties with their friends from school, but Susie, the two girls and I would also have our own celebration. The girls would get together on weekends, go to camp together, and spend holidays together. Alex was always at our house or our daughter at hers. They each of course had their own friends, but there is something special about your first real friend. Those two remained loyal to that friendship.

It's funny, because many times people described Alex as this perfect little angel. When my daughter and I heard that, we always had to laugh. We knew Alex from when she was a baby, and she was always causing mischief. I mean, she was never doing it in a hurtful way, but she loved to have a great time. She loved to laugh and tease. I have videos of her at the age of four singing and dancing and even mooning the camera. She was always the one who could look at something and realize what could be done to make it fun. To this day, there are things my daughter won't share with me about what Alex did or said, because Alex swore her to secrecy. I can only imagine, but I know it wasn't meant to be malicious. That wasn't Alex's way.

We knew that Alex had been having trouble with her knee. We knew she had corrective surgery but was still limping along. Then came the phone call. Susie asked, "Can your father get Alex in for an MRI? They're pretty sure she has cancer." Susie knew my father was a physician and that he did a lot of oncology work. I went right over to be with Susie, and when Billy came home, I gave him a hug. We were all in shock. That night I told my daughter, "You need to call Alex."

My daughter was asking me all kinds of questions. What I finally realized was that no matter how young you are or how old you are, when you hear someone has cancer, you think, "Oh well, they'll fix it and she'll be okay." That's what I thought and that's what my daughter thought. They'll fix it, and Alex will be as good as new. Not long after, I was talking to a woman in our neighborhood. My daughter and Alex often babysat for this woman's four children together. It was funny because Alex would get those kids all riled up and my daughter would be the one to calm them down. They were quite a team. So I told this woman, who happened to be a nurse, that Alex had cancer, that it was osteogenic sarcoma. I'll never forget the look on her face. It just dropped. That's when I realized how serious the situation really was.

So what do you do when your child's best friend has cancer? What do you do as a parent when your son or daughter may lose their first friend—their very best friend? You have the greatest concern for the person who is ill and for their family, but you also worry about your child and what they are going through.

First, you have to be able to read your own child's feelings and needs. Second, you have to walk a very fine line between being optimistic and full of hope and being blunt and honest about what may happen. It's not an easy line to walk. My husband and I went back and forth. He is more of a pragmatist, so he would say, "We have to tell her that Alex is probably not going to make it." I'd say, "No, we can't. There's always hope."

It is nice to have lots of friends, but I also believe that it's better to have five close friends that you can count on rather than 100 that drift in and out of your life. I tried to be that kind of friend for Susie, and my daughter was that kind of friend to Alex.

When illness strikes, it's important to remain the friend you have always been. Don't treat the person differently. In a strong relationship, the illness is certainly something that cannot be ignored, but it is the friend that is the priority. Your friend is not a cancer patient. Your friend is a patient with cancer. They are still the same friend. Sure, there are changes, but they are still the same person.

So when your child's best friend is faced with a life-threatening illness, it's especially important to know your child. It's important to walk the fine line between eternal hope and reality. It's important that as parents we support our sons and daughters in their efforts to sustain and honor that friendship. Many people can come in and out of your life depending on the circumstance, but true friends remain true friends.

You know, teenage daughters and their mothers are often at odds. My daughter and I still had our moments, but in a time when our friends faced adversity, my daughter and I gained respect for each other. We grew closer. I knew that whatever happened, my daughter was remaining a true friend to Alex, and I was remaining a true friend to Susie and Billy. Those are the kind of unconditional friendships we can hold onto for the rest of our lives.

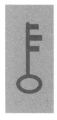

A life without people, without the same people day after day, people who belong to us, people who will be there for us, people who need us and whom we need in return, may be very rich in other things, but in human terms, it is no life at all.

Harold S. Kushner
Author, *When All You've Ever Wanted Isn't Enough*

Chemo

Bill

Journal Entry December 25, 1997:

I'm feeling better today. I haven't been too upset about my tumor and cancer ordeal. On Monday the 30th I will be in the hospital, because that's when I start chemotherapy. My leg still hurts from the biopsy, but the doctor said the pain will go away soon. Tomorrow I will have a bone scan. Then I can come home. The doctor will change my bandage on my leg and I think I can shower tomorrow. YEAH!

Alex

Alex, Susie and I met Dr. Main, the director of Pediatric Hematology and Oncology for William Beaumont Hospital in his office. He explained what was going to happen. There are standard protocols for treating osteogenic sarcoma. It's the same whether it is at Children's Hospital or Memorial Sloan-Kettering Cancer Center: 22 bouts of chemo. They put a Broviac catheter in the chest to administer the chemotherapy and other medications. Osteogenic sarcomas are very aggressive, and likewise, the treatment is very aggressive. They try to shrink the tumor with chemotherapy, surgically remove the cancer and follow that with another 15 chemotherapy treatments.

The chemotherapy treatments were much more than just going in for a day, then coming home. Each time, Alex had to be in the hospital for a week with a constant drip of chemo. The next week she would be doing okay, then the following week her blood count would drop, so she would end up back in the hospital for a blood transfusion. Because the chemotherapy attacks fast-growing tissue, it also kills white cells and red cells.

The patient's blood counts become so low that their immune system is dramatically weakened. To avoid infections they can't eat fresh fruit, be around flowers, or sometimes have visitors. Despite the transfusions and all the precautions, the patient's immune system is so ravaged, she still may get an infection requiring hospitalization for several more days.

When Alex was getting her chemo, she was not a happy camper. The side effects were so powerful, she actually threw up at home just thinking about going in for the next treatment. Once there, part of her "drip" would be an anti-nausea medication, but it didn't totally eliminate the nausea. The chemo ruined her appetite, and when offered food she usually responded, "I don't want to eat." It didn't take long before she became very thin.

One might think her friends would have avoided visiting that kind of uncomfortable situation, but not so. The kids never shied away. They would come and do their homework with her. They would talk and plan and gossip. Above all, her friends would listen. Alex was truly happy when they were there. Even on the days when she was not feeling well at all, her friends would just stay and sit. It wouldn't be uncommon to find one of the guys sleeping in a chair or one of her girlfriends next to her on the bed.

Alex was never alone in the hospital. Friends and family were constantly visiting, and we were always at her side. Susie and I took turns staying overnight. I think Alex felt very much taken care of…very much loved.

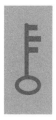

I suspect that the most basic and powerful way to connect to another person is to listen. Just listen. Perhaps the most important thing we give each other is our attention. And especially if it's given from the heart.

Rachel Naomi Remen, M.D.
Author, Kitchen Table Wisdom

Peds

Nurse Diane

After nursing school I went right into pediatrics. I've worked on "peds" for 20 years. It's the only branch of medicine I've ever worked, and it's all I've really wanted to do. It remains my passion. We have what's called primary nursing, which means as a nurse you have certain patients all the time. To cover different shifts and schedules, there were four assigned to take care of Alex when she was in the hospital. We liked to take care of our regular patients too, because then you are current on what is going on and you know exactly what happened the last time the patient was in for treatment.

I first met Alex right after she had her biopsy. We were getting her back into bed, and she was still a little groggy from the anesthesia. The first words out of her mouth were, "I don't want to lose my hair!" She was a beautiful young girl with long, flowing brown hair. And, of course, like any teenage girl would do, her immediate focus was on her looks. Her parents, on the other hand, were fretting about her health, her future, her very life.

At first I thought, this girl is going to be hard to handle. But then, when Alex got the news, she took it with an unusual calm. She was like, "All right. So let's fight this. What are we going to do?" Now, that is amazing for a teen and especially for a girl. Girls tend to be a bit more dramatic, but Alex faced the news with a warrior's face.

The best thing her parents did was to be open and tell her everything. I mean, sometimes we get these parents who have teenagers, and they want to conceal the truth. They tell us, "Don't tell them they have cancer. Just tell them they need this medicine to help them." So what are these kids to think when they start losing their hair? I remember a 9-year-old boy and his parents refused to tell him he had cancer. They just didn't understand. These kids know. They are not stupid. They see, they listen and they know what's going on. Parents like that mean well. They are afraid, too, and they are afraid their child is going to be upset if they are told the truth. Well of course the child will be upset, but overall, these young people do so much better when the parents tell them what's happening and how they are going to receive care and treatment.

There was another teenager I remember. She was the nastiest little girl to everyone, but I attribute a good part of that to the fact her parents never told her the truth. We all know that kids listen. Kids hear. Kids know. How does that make them feel when the ones they should be able to trust the most keep them in the dark? Living in the dark leaves the patient living in fear, and with kids, their fears can be worse than reality. If they can't trust what their parents are telling them, they begin imagining all sorts of horrible things. What's the old saying? "Nothing's worse than the fear of the unknown."

Alex's parents kept her informed. Everything was discussed in front of her, and Alex was an active part of every decision. I believe that gave her some sense of control in a world that for her and every other cancer patient is out of their control. Not only did Alex know and participate in the decisions about her situation and treatment, she would help other youngsters on the floor. For example, when one of the other patients was going in for her first chemo, Alex shared with her what she had experienced. When it's the first time, you don't know what to expect, but Alex had been there. She would talk to the other patients about the sick feelings they would experience and the anti-nausea medicine options. She would say, "Well, this is what works for me." And just like a big sister, she would go on, "You know this is what we're going to do."

Those were the kinds of moments that made us take special notice of Alex. I mean, when acting as a primary nurse, you work with patients and their families so much you can't help but develop personal relationships. In Alex's case, each time she was going to be admitted the other primary care nurses and I would actually stand there fighting over her. You know, it was like: "I get her. No, I get her. No, I get her." It was all said in a fun way, but it typified how we felt about Alex. She was always so positive and so caring. It made you want to be around her.

Alex didn't dwell on the medical challenges of the present but looked forward to the future. In fact, she had taken up photography, and she talked about all the things she wanted to take pictures of. She told me, "When I get out of here, I'll come over and take pictures of your kids."

What has stayed with me to this day was one of the things she said. I guess it stuck out because most teenagers have out-of-sight aspirations, and for the most part that's good. I mean, most teenagers feel like they are going to recreate the world or be president or a singing star on MTV. It was during one of the times Alex was pretty sick and not doing well. I wanted to get her mind on something else, so I asked her what she wanted to do with her life. She paused, and then replied, "I want to be a soccer mom. I want to have kids and drive them all around."

"I just want to be a soccer mom."

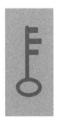

It is when things go hardest, when life becomes the most trying, that there is the greatest need for having a fixed goal. When few comforts come from without, it is all the more necessary to have a fount to draw from within.

B.C. Forbes
Financial journalist and author

Dating Alex

Friend Jason

Journal Entry February 12, 1998:

Today was one of the worst days. I threw up for about an hour. My friend, my grandpa and grandma and the rabbi came to see me.

Alex

Even though I chose not to see or call Alex for months, when we began talking again she opened up to me. It was in those early days, right after her diagnosis, that I ever saw her fearful of anything. She told me she was scared. She was scared that cancer was going to kill her. We had this whole conversation about death. It was intense. She cried, and I promised her repeatedly that she would be fine. I promised her she was not going to die. I believed she would be fine.

I went to Alex's house every day after school. We talked on the phone just about every night sometimes until 4 or 5 in the morning. Alex was having treatments, and everything seemed about the same to me. She still looked the same. She still acted the same, and we were able to go out and do the same kinds of things teenagers did. One time, early in her treatments, I went to see her at the hospital. To me she looked fine. She looked like the same exact girl.

At first there was nothing between us romantically. Alex and I had become close friends. We enjoyed hanging out together, and we spent countless hours talking on the phone. It wasn't long before my friends started asking me, "Do you like Alex? Are you starting to get feelings for her?" I was always like,

"No. I don't like Alex." Well…you know how teenage guys are. Privately I had this vision of Alex and me as girlfriend and boyfriend. I saw this whole cancer thing passing and being the thing that brought us back together. I would be the one to help her through her ordeal, and when it was over we would date. One day we would look back and laugh about the whole thing. How romantic is that?

Things started to change. One day I called her and Alex says, "Some of my hair fell out this morning." I'm like, "Oh, don't worry." She says, "No, I've got to go to the salon today, and they are going to cut it really short." I'm still like, "Don't worry. It will be fine. It will all grow back." I'm starting to ask myself, "Wow. What's going on here? What's with this cancer thing? What am I really feeling for Alex?"

One day I was talking to a couple of Alex's friends, and they start talking about me taking her on a "real date" for Valentine's Day. They're like, "Yeah. Do it. She wants you to do it." It didn't take too much encouragement. I asked Alex out on a Valentine's date and she accepted.

I got some flowers for her and went to pick her up for the date. It was a bit weird for me, because here I'm out with a girl about my age, and she couldn't really walk very well. She had a cane and her hair was really, really short. Still I'm thinking, "Alex is really pretty. She still looks good to me. If this is the worst it gets, I can deal with it." The date went fine and before the night was over, we were making out. "Wow. This is really cool. We really care about each other, and by the summer this cancer thing is going to be done."

But it wasn't done. Things didn't seem to be getting better. Every time we went out her parents were like, "You have to be really careful. If she falls and hurts her leg, it will be horrible." I'm thinking this really sucks, but I'm also still thinking this is a temporary thing. Yet, for a teenage boy, it was a bit much. It wasn't long after that Alex was over at my house. We were in the basement, holding hands and having this difficult, gut-wrenching discussion. Alex tells me, "Look, I would like to date you, but I can't do that right now. My life is just too crazy what with all these treatments and everything." Alex had always been very direct, so I figured this is the way she wanted it. I wanted to be her boyfriend, but I have to admit, it was getting pretty strange for this high school senior. I mean, I had lots of things I wanted to do. This was my last year at North Farmington, and I wanted to celebrate and do the things seniors do.

Alex and I continued to talk and be friends, but I went on with my life too. I mean, this was what we agreed upon, right? Alex was sick, but I wasn't. We still were close. We still talked just about every night. Every time before saying goodbye, I'd say, "I love you." Alex would answer, "I love you too." I still wanted to be there for her, but now things were different.

I went on spring break and met this girl. We came back and began dating. I chose not to tell Alex.

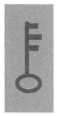

No one lives forever; therefore, death is not the issue. Life is. Death is not a failure. Not choosing to take on the challenge of life is.

Bernie S. Siegel, M.D.
Author, *Love, Medicine & Miracles*

A Video for the Phlebotomist

Sandy, Phlebotomist

I'm not a doctor. I'm not a nurse. I'm a phlebotomist. I'm the one responsible for collecting blood for testing through finger pokes and arm draws.

Back in 1980 I applied and accepted a position in phlebotomy at Beaumont Hospital. During my years there, I met Dr. Charles (Chuck) Main in pediatric oncology because my 18-month-old son was diagnosed with hemophilia. As we cared for my son's needs, we developed a relationship with the pediatric oncology team. In time, I became aware of an opening for a pediatric phlebotomist. I was lucky enough to get the job, and it's a decision and career choice I would never change. I think of all the kids I've met and all the lives I have had the opportunity to touch. Twenty-five years later I'm going to the weddings and baby showers of the patients I served. They thank me, but in the end, I'm the one who feels fortunate to have met and known them.

I see patients that are diagnosed, but, for the most part, they don't know what they are up against. I do. In my role, I see the kids so much. I see them more often than the doctors and the nurses. The kids come in to get their blood tested from one to three times a week, and, for some, even more often. They can get into a situation where we don't know exactly what's going on with their platelets, their hemoglobin, or if they are going to get transfused. They can be checked one day and be borderline, so there is a need for them to come back the next day. Sometimes the weekly testing can continue for years.

My goal is to make them comfortable coming in for their finger pokes, or arm draws or whatever. I try to add some fun to their visits. If I can do that, it's going to make it easier on the child and on the entire family. Sometimes, the patients, especially those in their teens, are understandably very angry and bitter. I know that bitterness is going to make treatment rough on them and on their families. Those are tough ones, but you just start working to make it better a little at a time.

We start playing games like, "What's your platelet count this time?" Or, "Who can guess the closest?" For example, we would have candy for the kids and over time we would find the newest treats and patient's favorites. We have some connections, so sometimes we could get things like concert tickets for the older kids. We even have every kind of Band-Aid you could imagine. I'm telling you, when I have a 14- or 15-year-old boy there, and I tell him to close his eyes while I apply the Band-Aid, and he opens his eyes to see one with guitars...well, I usually get a chuckle. A small reaction like that can be very positive.

Sometimes the treatment can be heavy duty like a bone marrow or a spinal tap. It's important for us to be sensitive. The kids have every right to be upset. They have every right not to be there, but there they are. I never belittle it. I never tell them it's no big deal. We would have special prizes for them, thanks to gifts and fundraisers from the community and companies such as K-Mart and Best Buy. For the older ones, prizes such as a phone cards can help the kids keep in touch with their friends. The giving and support of the private and business communities is so awesome and makes such a difference!

The teenagers that come in are very apprehensive. They are typically angry. They are very, very angry. They are in what they feel is the prime of their life. Now they are going to lose their hair. Now they can't participate in their favorite activities. They have gone through test after test after test, and what am I going to do? I'm going to poke them one more time. So, the starting point is a challenging one. It's a matter of developing a relationship over time and earning their trust. With teenagers, it's always a struggle.

Alex was a teenager, and she was skeptical too, but there was something about her. She just seemed to take it all in. I'd describe her as a whirlwind. She was always a whirlwind when she came in. She would hang out in my office with some of the other kids waiting for their time to see the doctor. She would want to know what was going on with everyone. She would want to know about me and about my family. She would be telling me about her life and about things like the music she was into. She loved James Taylor and Cat Stevens. In a way I thought that was a bit odd for her age, but she was quite diverse in her likes and dislikes. She was also big time in love with the new group, the Barenaked Ladies.

While my goal was to lift the spirits of the patients, Alex was the one to lift my spirits. There were times I was having a rough day and I'm like, "Whoops, Alex is coming in at 11:00. I wonder what will be up with her today. I wonder what stories she will have to tell." What was amazing about Alex was her concern for others. She would talk to someone in the waiting room who was having a bad day. She developed friendships with the other patients and would visit them. She would leave notes with me for other patients. She would say things like, "When you see her, give her my number. I haven't heard from her. Tell her to call me." And, unlike the typical teenager, I never, ever heard her say anything angry about what she was going through.

We developed a close relationship. Sometimes she would even call me late at night just to chat. There was nothing wrong in particular, she just wanted to talk. We were both big *Saturday Night Live* fans, so we would talk about the guest and the skits, and we both enjoyed movies, so we would talk about that. There were also times she just couldn't sleep at night and wanted to talk about more important things. It was almost like she had things that she needed to take care of—things that she needed to resolve like difficulties she was experiencing with a friendship. She talked to me about things that were important to her. She worried about her mom and dad. She worried about her family and her friends. Interestingly enough, she never spoke to me about her prognosis. That was one of the things that was so moving about the video she sent me when I was off work for surgery. She plays a Cat Stevens song on it.

The video opened with, "Get well soon, please. Miss you. Here are some pictures so you know how I looked before January." Her message is followed by a series of photos. Alex was so young and healthy—so full of life. As she turned the photos one at a time, Cat Stevens sang, "...Look at me. Take your time. Think of everything you've got...I know I have to go away. I know I have to go."

Later on in the video, Alex shares, "I got my blood poked today. It was weird. Normally when you are not there, I know you will be back the next day, but today I really missed you. I'm like worried about your surgery. I don't know how it went. I don't what the surgery was or anything. I just hope you are feeling well. So to cheer us both up I thought we'd sing our song. I'll start and you can join in. I'll be your crying shoulder...."

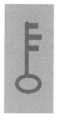

Those who have the gift of inspiration exude something that's difficult to pin down intellectually, yet is undeniably recognizable in how we feel in their presence.

Wayne W. Dyer, Ph.D.
Author, *Inspiration: Your Ultimate Calling*

Skip Metastasis

Susie

Journal Entry April 22, 1998:

Today was a roller coaster, worrying about my baby's upcoming operation and being uplifted by calls and e-mail messages of support. When you came home for the evening, I told you that Rabbi Spectre called to say that half of his meeting in New York was spent "talking about Alex Graham."

You turned around, smiled and said, "I feel so loved."

Dad

They began giving Alex chemotherapy in December and continued through March. The treatments were taking their toll, and the side effects were powerful. Alex would throw up in the bathroom taking a bath while she was getting ready to go to the hospital for a treatment. Just thinking about chemo was enough to make her throw up. It was tough.

The tumor was not shrinking, and Alex was feeling something up in her groin area. She felt—I don't know—a swelling or something. Dr. Irwin checked it and called it a skip metastasis. The doctor said, "Here are the choices. You get your leg amputated, you live." Remarkably Alex was okay with it. I mean she wasn't like, "Oh, my God, my leg!" Somehow she took it in stride.

We tried to keep calm in front of her, but for me just thinking of that leg being amputated was like a death in itself. I felt that way. I mean, here is this beautiful girl, my beautiful daughter. She was 5-foot-7, long blond hair and blue eyes. She was beautiful inside and out. Just the thought of her losing her leg, her hair, her freedom. I was sick for her. It was devastating to know this was going to happen to her.

I did everything I could not to project those feelings to her. I cried a lot when she wasn't around. I'd allow myself to cry, mostly in the car when I was by myself, because there wasn't a place or often the time. Here's the thing: I could find a moment to cry, but it wasn't so much the crying as it was going with red, swollen eyes to see Alex or meet with someone. So it was tough. It was really tough to let my feelings go.

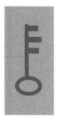

It may be that when we no longer know what to do, we have come to our real work, and when we no longer know which way to go, we have begun our real journey.

Wendell Berry
American author

Two Baldies

Aunt Elaine

Journal Entry April 23, 1990.

The doctor called to see if you could come to see a patient who had her hip and leg amputated. "She even rollerblades now." She has a new leg from a place in Flint, the best he has ever seen.

Dad

My family lived in the small town of Belleville, Michigan. When I turned 16 and a sophomore in high school, my brother Billy was born. He was so cute and so much younger that I took every opportunity to spoil him.

After I finished high school, I met my future husband. We decided to marry and make our home in Belleville as well. When my brother Billy grew up, he met the love of his life, Susie. The two of them traveled quite a bit, so, when they had their children, the kids would often come to stay with us. We had a small pool the kids enjoyed, and my husband had a riding lawn mower the boys liked to drive. David, Robbie and Alex thought visiting their aunt and uncle was great fun. They said they would rather stay with us in Belleville than go to Disneyland. I guess they liked visiting us almost as much as we enjoyed having them.

Alex was this bubbly, energetic, young girl. She was a bit mischievous and had this infectious sense of humor. When we found out she had cancer, we were just devastated. I remember going to Beaumont Hospital to see her. She was just beginning the long string of chemotherapy treatments. There in the hospital bed laid this child—so full of potential with her long brown hair,

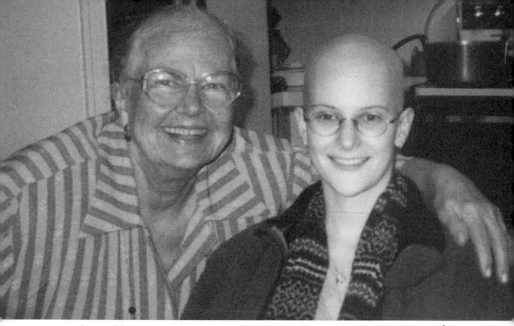

Alex and her aunt celebrate life while enduring the effects of chemotherapy.

crisp white socks and one-of-a-kind smile. My heart ached for her and I guess I was feeling guilty. It wasn't fair. I was 70, still working, and a picture of health. Why her? Why not me?

Not long after, it was me. I was diagnosed with colon cancer. Pretty soon Alex and I had both lost our hair from the chemo. I've got a picture of us together. I call it "the two baldies." Despite our illness, we still enjoyed our time together. Alex's sense of humor shone through as we looked in the mirror and giggled about our hairless heads.

She could easily have been filled with self pity, but she wasn't. Through it all Alex was unbelievably brave, unbelievably strong. Yet what amazed me was something more than her courage and strength. She was going through what no one should ever have to go through, and somehow this teenager remained so caring, so supportive, so concerned about others. At times I wondered if I could make it through the day. Alex was more like, "What can I do for you? How can I make you happy?" She sent me cards to lift my spirits, and her simple words still speak to me today.

I hope you are feeling better from the surgery. I especially hope they can take care of the mass easily. I know we can get through this if we tell ourselves we can. I love you, and I promise everything will be better soon. Cheer up. I'm here for you.
Love,
Alex

My niece and I were just a couple of baldies, but I was 70 and she was only 16 years old.

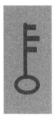

To send a letter is a good way to go somewhere without anything but your heart.

Phyllis Theroux
American essayist, columnist and author

I Didn't Want to Deal with It

David

A blood and platelet plan based on Alex's treatment schedule was set up to coordinate the "directed" blood donations with the Red Cross. So many people wanted to donate. There were over fifty volunteers from one company alone. Some people were actually upset that they couldn't donate directly to Alex, because of blood type or iron deficiency. In the end, there was a key group of about five main donors for blood and about three for platelets.

Susie

You get scared when people are sick. You don't know what to do. I was her older brother, and yet I was trying to stay away. I know it doesn't make sense, but that's the way it was. Maybe I was immature. Maybe I was just a bad brother, or maybe it was normal for a young guy my age. I can't say exactly why, but I tried to withdraw as much as possible. I just didn't want to deal with it.

I was working full time, and it seemed like Alex was always in the hospital. That meant I didn't see her or mom or dad that much. For the most part it was easy to stay isolated, but then there were times it was impossible, like when Alex was home. Her bedroom was right next to mine, so I could hear when she was awake at night. Sometimes it was like she didn't sleep at all. I could hear her moving around or talking on the phone. Sometimes I could hear her crying. I didn't know exactly what to do. I figured the best thing for me was to stay out of the way and be there to help when asked.

My sister and I didn't spend much time together. I regret

that now. We were almost eight years apart in age, and she liked hanging out with her friends. I did take her to the movies now and then, and I won't ever forget the last film we went to see. *Patch Adams* was showing at the Star Movie Complex, and Alex wasn't feeling well. She was having a real tough time. I'll never watch that movie again, but not because the movie was bad. It's just that it brings back too many memories, too many feelings.

There was one way I was able to help. We had to get a list of people together to give blood and platelets. Alex would need them after chemo when her white blood counts were low. The donor couldn't be a family member, because donations from family members had to be saved for a bone marrow transplant. But get this: Because I was adopted, I could donate blood platelets right away. Even more amazing was that I had the same blood type as Alex!

I'd have to describe the blood platelets donation process as the worst. I would go to the Red Cross apheresis clinic, and the procedure would take an hour or more. They would sit me in a chair and put one huge needle in each arm. I mean, these needles looked enormous! It hurt so badly. They tell you beforehand not to drink a lot. I didn't think much about it until I realized that once you start the process you can't leave the chair. You're not even allowed to move your arms, and if you've got to go to the bathroom, well…too bad. You just had to wait until the process was over.

I guess through it all I was scared, and I was mad. My little sister was sick and I didn't know what to do. It wasn't fair that she was going through this, and it didn't seem like anyone could stop it, not even the doctors. Isn't it funny? I was the big brother, and I was scared. Then there was Alex. She was a teenager battling cancer, and she was stronger than all of us.

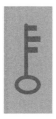

The emotions are not always subject to reason…but they are always subject to action. When thoughts do not neutralize an undesirable emotion, action will.

William James
Psychologist and philosopher

The Amputation

Friends Sarah and Illana

Journal Entry April 24, 1998:

Well, it's 12:36 A.M. on Friday morning and I have so many thoughts going through my head. Today will soon be the beginning of something new. Even though I will be losing something, I will also be gaining strength and a hell of a lot of power. Losing my leg will be extremely hard for me, but I know that my life will still carry on.

Alex

A friend of ours had a part-time job working at a local specialty cake bakery. Alex and I would go there to hang out with her while she was working. We would sneak behind the counter and help her make boxes for the cakes. Of course, we always had to taste a sample or two of the cake of the day. That day, Alex had a doctor's appointment, so the plan was for the three of us to meet at the bakery when she was finished.

Months before, when Alex first told us about the cancer, there were tears. Since then she had shown us her confidence and determination to beat the disease, and we shared in that confidence. Through all the treatments, she displayed the same old energy and sense of humor we loved to be around. I always thought, "She's going to fight it, and she's going to be fine." I never thought anything bad was going to happen.

When Alex arrived at the bakery we greeted her as always. "Hey, Alex! How did it go? You have just got to try this new cake!"

"Guys, I need to tell you something. I'm going to have my leg amputated. They said it would be best for me. It will make me live, so it's just what I have to do."

We didn't know what to say. We couldn't believe what we were hearing. The thought of her losing her leg was unimaginable, and there she stood talking like she was okay with it. Alex was clearly so much stronger than the rest of us. Looking back, I realize it was her strength and attitude that got her, me and everyone else through it all.

It was that way from the beginning of our friendship, too. I remember as little kids Alex and I went to summer camp at Willoway. For me it was the first time away from home for more than a day or two. It was for two whole weeks! At that age when you are homesick, two weeks can seem like forever. Then there was Alex. She never felt homesick. She was the strong one, and there she was, day after day, making me laugh and trying to cheer me up.

I was also the shy one, but around Alex, I became less fearful of acting out. After Willoway and camps to follow, we would entertain ourselves by dressing up in crazy clothes and singing and dancing to the camp songs we had learned. Sometimes our moms would videotape us putting on our little shows. Years later we would watch the videos together and end up laughing until we cried.

There were tears before Alex's amputation too, but not from Alex. Even the night before the operation, she insisted we paint her toenails to impress the doctor. She wanted everything to "look okay." Alex also wrote little messages all over her bad leg with different color markers like, "Take this one." Her strength and sense of humor shone through at times when we were at

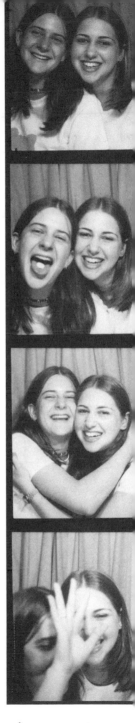

Alex cherished her friendships and enjoyed every moment.

our weakest. The day she was to have her leg removed, a bunch of friends were with her before she was wheeled off to the operating room. The doctor had stopped by to see how she was doing and talk to her one more time. The tension of the moment made it hard for me to breathe, but just like when we were kids at camp, Alex knew when I needed her the most. As the doctor was leaving the room, Alex thrust out her hand to shake the doctor's, and in her confident, raspy voice she goes, "Good luck, Dr. Irwin! Make sure you do the right leg."

The doctor smiled, and we all started to crack up. We needed the emotional release, and right on cue, there was Alex to put a smile on our face. Another door was closing on her world, yet she reminded us that laughter and hope were there for the taking. That was the last time we saw Alex before the amputation. Her leg was lost, but she never lost any part of who she was as a person.

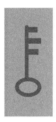

A sense of humor can help you overlook the unattractive, tolerate the unpleasant, cope with the unexpected, and smile through the unbearable.

Rabbi Moshe Waldoks
Spiritual leader, author and humorist

I Take Care of Zebras

Ronald B. Irwin, M. D.

Journal Entry April 24, 1998:

You came out of surgery in pain, but by late afternoon you were doing better. About 8:20 p.m. I went out to get some of your belongings from the minivan. As I returned to pediatrics I heard, "Pediatric CPR to room 4727!" That was your room! When I got there the room was full of nurses and doctors. Mom was in the hallway crying. They had a tube down your throat and an oxygen mask on your face. The head resident was trying to calm you down. You said, "You're not a real doctor! I want Dr. Irwin!"

Dad

I'm an orthopedic oncologist. I take care of zebras. What do I mean by that? In medical school we are taught a year of what's referred to as "hoofs and horses." In other words, if you hear the hoofs of horses look for horses. You are taught to assess the patient by thinking of the most common thing that could be wrong first. You are not supposed to think first of the odd things. My specialty is different. In my role I am looking for the "zebra." I am looking for the unusual and untypical. I have the advantage of looking back and knowing what has happened prior to the patient coming to me. While the average orthopedic surgeon is going to see one osteogenic sarcoma in her or his whole life, between new patients and follow-ups, I see four a day. I take care of people with musculoskeletal tumors, bone cancer and soft-tissue cancer. There are only three of us in the entire state that do this all day, and that's pretty much been my life since 1978.

When Alex first came to me she showed a very subtle X-ray presentation. At the time MRI was fairly new and not readily available. It seemed apparent to me that she probably had a cancer of the femur bone, so we did a biopsy. The typical treatment for someone with that condition would be chemotherapy for two to four months followed by a surgical procedure and then another eight months of chemo. The extent of the disease is very important. There are osteogenic sarcomas and there are osteogenic sarcomas. They are graded one through four or one through three. Hers was a very high grade. These days we normally try to save the leg, even if the whole femur is gone. We substitute a cadaver bone or metal, but there are times, like in her case, when amputation may be the only alternative. It may sound a bit callous, but I don't mind doing the amputation if I think doing so gives us a chance to cure the patient.

One of the rewards of my job is the relationship you build with your patients. You try to save their lives or at least improve their quality of life. You build such a bond that you actually fall in love with some of them. I know that might sound weird, but Alex was one of those patients. She loved me, and I loved her. She was uniquely intelligent and highly interested in this whole phenomena and how it impacted the patients and everyone in the hospital. She was somehow at ease with her illness. She understood it, and spent most of her time fighting it and not whining about it. She wanted to know all the details. She wanted to know what you were doing, why you were doing it and how it was going to be done.

Alex wasn't just interested in matters that related to her condition. She took interest in those around her. She cared about her family, her friends, the other patients and those who provided her medical care and attention. In my profession you spend a lot of time with your patients and their families. You develop personal relationships and mutual respect. Alex and I had that, and we had fun too. For example, I always got a kick out of her when it came to my motorcycle. If she thought I had been out on my Harley, she would give me hell. She'd say, "You can't do that, Dr. Irwin! I need you!"

For Alex's condition, a hip-disarticulation was the best chance we had of saving her life. The morning of her amputation

I came in to see her and, to no one's surprise, she was giving me last-minute instructions. Patients often direct a lot of anger at their physicians, especially those who may be about to remove their limb, but not Alex. She shook my hand and said, "Good luck, Doctor," but she said something more. She also told me, "I love you, Doctor Irwin," and I said, "You know, Alex, I love you too."

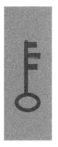 It is not how you deal with what is expected and hoped for in your life that ultimately defines and elevates you as a human being. Rather, it is how you Interact with the unexpected, how you brave the unanticipated, how you navigate through the unforeseen and emerge, transformed and reborn, on the other side.

Barbara De Angelis, Ph.D.
Author, *How Did I Get Here?*

The Encounter

Grandmother Scheinker

Journal Entry April 27, 1998:

The physical therapist came to see you today in the hospital. You were able to get up and take a few steps by yourself. The doctor changed your dressing. It was his "best job." The stitches appear to be such that they will be covered by your bathing suit.

The doctors reported that they spoke to experts from New York's Memorial Sloan-Kettering Hospital. They suspect that you are not absorbing the methotrexate well. We will likely fly to New York in a couple of weeks to check it out. We're considering having your lung surgery there.

Dad

When I was born my family lived in an area on the east side of Detroit known as Westminster. It was a very ethnic neighborhood, much like a little New York. We lived in an area where there were a lot of children. We lived in flats. Families were on all sides of you, and kids were always playing in the streets. But we were also in an area that had elements of the notorious Purple Gang. Growing up we were always warned, "Be careful. Don't go past the corner!"

Later our family moved to what was called the Dexter area. It was very much the same. We were always fortunate to be surrounded by friends and family. That's where I met my husband, Sidney. I was 14 and he was 15.

Sidney and our granddaughter, Alex, had a very special relationship. Alex was so much like my Susie was as a child: very outgoing and loved to sing and dance. Now Alex and my Sidney loved to tease each other. Alex would say, "You want a cat, don't you, Grandpa?" With a smirk he would shake his head and groan, "No, I don't want a cat." She'd chime back, "Yes, Grandpa, you want that cat!" They'd both laugh, and so it went.

Watching Alex and her family go through so much was heartbreaking. Alex was so brave. We couldn't know what she was going through, but I think we all suffered right with her. Back and forth to the hospital they went...back and forth and back and forth. Sidney would say, "Why her? Why didn't it happen to me? I've lived my life. I've lived a full life. Why must this happen to my Alex?"

Something happened that I will never forget. I call it an encounter.

I once worked as a volunteer for Meals on Wheels. I delivered meals to a high-rise residential complex known as the Highland Towers. At the time, Alex was back in the hospital recovering from her amputation. Well, I was standing in the Highland Towers elevator consumed by my thoughts... wondering how Alex was doing...wondering how this could all be happening. Suddenly I realized I was standing next to a tall man who was leaning on a crutch. He was missing a leg.

I looked up, and I said, "Oh, my God! My granddaughter just had her leg amputated." And we started to talk. He said, "Would you mind if I went to see her. I'm a preacher, and I'd like to meet her." I told him she was over at William Beaumont Hospital.

So later that day, into Alex's room walked this big, tall African American man with one leg. Alex and Susie didn't know who he was or why he was there. He began to explain, "I met your grandmother on an elevator. We talked, and I'm here to share something with you." Alex looked at him in amazement and exclaimed, "I know you! I saw you in the restaurant!" Apparently just days before going into the hospital, Alex and her friends had gone to dinner at a restaurant in Royal Oak. While they were there, this man walked in and Alex noticed that he was missing his leg. She watched him and wondered what life might hold for her. She never mentioned it to anyone.

His visit to the hospital was meant to give her confidence.

He told her, "Look at me. I'm getting around. I'm active. I'm living a full life and sharing my message."

Later, when Alex and Susie shared what had happened, they described him as an angel, and maybe he was. Call it what you want. I call it an encounter.

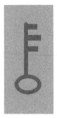

Choose to love and make others happy, and your life will change, because you will find happiness and love in the process. The first step toward inner peace is to decide to give love not receive it.

Bernie S. Siegel, M.D.
Author, *Love, Medicine & Miracles*

Friends

Susie

Journal Entry.

My friends came and brought me cards, candy, gum, magazines and an album. I love everyone, and it made me feel good to see who stood by me when I needed them most.

Alex

Her friends...the kids...they never stopped coming. Never. That is a story in itself. They literally rallied around her and never left her alone. Watching these young people demonstrate such unwavering loyalty to our daughter was an inspiration and brought comfort to us all.

Even during Alex's illness, her friends still looked to her as a leader. "Hey, what do you want to do, Alex? Where do you want to go?" And they would take Alex with them everywhere. I mean, no hair, a little stocking cap, one leg...they just didn't care about that. It was unbelievable for kids that age. They even took her to the National Hockey League Stanley Cup Playoffs.

In one case, a male friend asked Alex to go to a local carnival. Amusement parks and rides were among her favorite things, so she wasn't going to let the loss of her hair and her leg stop her from living life. While at the carnival, a young boy came up to her friend and said, "Hi, you were my camp counselor." Then he asked, "What happened to your girlfriend's leg?" In a nonchalant voice Alex's friend responded, "Vietnam." Later, when we heard their account of what happened, we all found ourselves laughing. Given the circumstance, the response was kind of funny. I mean, what do you say in a situation like that? We all had to laugh.

About the same time there was a popular song, "I'm Too Sexy." Alex had a great sense of humor and that shone through even as she battled cancer. She liked to put on a show for us and her friends. I think it was part of her way to deal with the tension and help put others at ease. So, after her amputation, it was vintage Alex for her to sing, "I'm too sexy. I'm too sexy for my leg. I'm too sexy. I'm too sexy for my leg."

It would have been easy for Alex to become totally self-absorbed in her world and in spending time with her friends. I mean, who would have blamed her? Yet, with the help and support of those friends, Alex chose to befriend others dealing with pain, discomfort and loneliness. She went with her youth group to visit a nursing home. Before going, she insisted we pick up some large-print books for her to share with the residents. Her friends told us later that while they were there, Alex actually got out of her own wheelchair and had one of the patients get in. On one leg, she hobbled and pushed the nursing home resident about for a stroll.

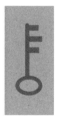

Believe, when you are most unhappy, that there is something for you to do in the world. So long as you can sweeten another's pain, life is not in vain.

Helen Keller
Author and activist

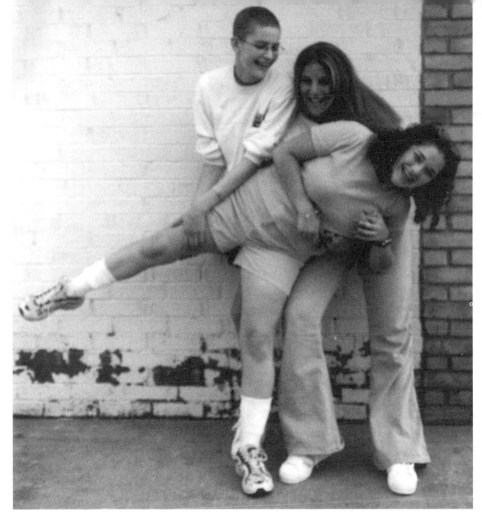

With the support of her friends, Alex finds ways to smile despite losing her leg.

It's All About Attitude

Thomas M. Bremer, Prosthetist

Journal Entry April 28, 1998:

Today they wanted you to walk for the first time on one leg and crutches. They were hoping you could make it 10 feet, but you surprised everybody by walking 200! The physical therapist kept saying, "Awesome! Awesome!" All of the nurses were watching you. I noticed one crying some tears of joy. I have never been so proud of you.

Dad

At the prosthetics clinic we fit all levels of amputees, all ages and all sizes. Each and every prosthetic is completely customized. The process starts with either a computer image or a plaster cast of the person's remaining limb. From the cast we pour a mold. Then we sculpt the mold to create weight-bearing areas, which avoid placing unnecessary pressure on the bones or irritating sensitive areas. Prototype testing is conducted to get the socket fitted comfortably, and then we address the alignment of the knees, feet and components.

Once the person is up and ambulating or walking well and all the alignment is correct, the foot and knee choices are made. From there we are able to finish off the prosthesis out of lightweight epoxies and carbon-fiber composites. The last step is cosmetics. We will actually take tracings of the individual's other limbs. We make a mirror image so we can shape the prosthetic. We match skin tone and spray on what's called a skin coat.

In Alex's case we were dealing with a hip disarticulation. That is the highest level of prosthetic we create. It gets very involved because you have a mechanical hip joint, a mechanical knee joint, and a mechanical foot joint. Every joint in the lower limb comes into play mechanically. Basically we had to sculpt a socket that she could actually slide into, close around her waist and sit in. In order to sit, she would have to bend her hip forward so the hip joint would bend. Then she would be able to sit right on the prosthesis. It was really involved.

I've been in the prosthetic field for almost 30 years. I've seen a lot of different levels and worked with some very talented prosthetists. To be the best it takes a mixture of art and science, and you need a lot of both. Some people think with technology, you should be able to do anything, but you have to remember the socket is just a fitting. If it isn't shaped properly or fitted around the anatomy just right, it doesn't work. Then there are the joints themselves. Take for example the knee joint. They range from simple hinged devices with a weight-activated brake, to hydraulic and air-driven pneumatic. The joints are made of very lightweight materials such as titanium or an aluminum alloy.

Alex started with a fairly simple hydraulic knee joint. The thing about Alex was that she was still very ill when she came to us, and it takes 60 percent more oxygen to walk with a leg prosthesis than to walk with two healthy legs. Consider the oxygen consumption, then add to that the fact Alex was still going through chemotherapy.

The truly amazing thing about Alex was that she always arrived at the clinic ready to work. I mean she just worked and worked and never complained. To be honest, it was inspiring just to see someone with her limited strength stand up. The staff noticed it from the minute she entered the front door. We knew Alex was coming in with a positive attitude, ready to take on the day. She had the kind of spirit everyone was attracted to and respected.

Some people won't use a hip prosthesis at all, because it requires so much energy and effort. For Alex, we knew it was going to be extremely difficult, yet she was determined to succeed. Keep in mind that in addition to the physical demands, there is the whole emotional side of acceptance. Reckoning with this poor substitute for a real limb takes a long time; sometimes years. It begins with a shocking reality that sets in when an individual first puts on their prosthesis. They are thinking, "I'm in shape. I'm athletic. I can do this." Then they put on the prosthesis and go, "Oh my God! All these joints are so different, and they're not attached!" It takes a long time to master a hip prosthesis, even for someone who is in otherwise excellent condition.

Young Alex wasn't in good health. She was immersed in an all-out battle with cancer, yet when she came to our clinic she gave it her all. She first walked using the parallel bars, and eventually she walked independently. She had major pain issues, but she proved she could do it. You know, I have had clients in their 50s who have undergone an amputation. They have adequate physical ability and strength, but they think, "Well, it's over. I'll never do this." Then there are people in their 90s who

Tom Bremer fits Alex with her prosthetic leg.

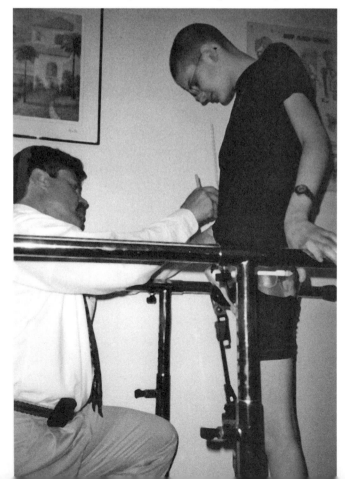

have an amputation, and within a year they are back on their feet and out working in their garden.

It's all about attitude, and Alex exhibited the kind of attitude that never said quit. For me, working with her was one of those times when my job was truly a gift...a gift I got paid to do. Most people undergoing chemotherapy would have been flat on their back but not Alex. Seeing how she pushed forward in the face of adversity, I would have done anything for her. You name it. For Alex I would have done whatever she needed.

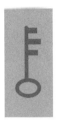

…everything can be taken from a man but one thing: the last of human freedoms—to choose one's attitude in any given set of circumstances, to choose one's own way.

Viktor Frankl
Author, *Man's Search for Meaning*

Physical Therapy

Kimberly, Physical Therapist

Journal Entry April 29, 1998:

It looks like you will have three legs; one for school/work, one for biking and sports and one for dressing fancy.

Dad

I have been a physical therapist for over 10 years. In 1998 I was in charge of coordinating a prosthetic and orthopedic clinic at the William Beaumont Hospital outpatient facility. That is where I first met Alex and her mother Susie. They came in to talk about the type of therapy Alex would be undertaking. I remember it was in July, about three months after her amputation.

Due to the extent of Alex's bone cancer and type of amputation, the prosthesis she required was extremely cumbersome. It was the type that on average required up to 180 percent of the effort for each step taken compared to someone with two functional limbs. Compound that with a young girl who was battling the side effects of chemotherapy, medications, transfusions, blood draws and injections. She was also very thin, so the prosthesis was extremely uncomfortable against her bony little pelvis. It was an unbelievably difficult situation. One would think these challenges would add up to one miserable and difficult patient to work with; a patient who would be discouraged, sad, complaining and whining. Many patients in otherwise good health who suffer that kind of amputation would have chosen not to ambulate with a prosthesis at all.

Well, that was absolutely not the case with Alex. She was a

joy. She did not complain, and not once did I hear her mutter the words, "Why me?" Instead, Alex focused on functioning normally and doing as much as she possibly could. My priority was to get her physically strong, so she could experience life as she desired. I also wanted her to be comfortable and emotionally adjusted to her situation. Her parents mirrored that thinking. They wanted Alex to experience all life had to offer, so they did things like going up north on vacation and taking her for a hot air balloon ride. In short, life went on.

Alex's progress physically was in some ways limited and in others phenomenal. Given the chemotherapy, the injections and their side effects, there were days when we could do very little, but Alex was always willing to try. There was even one day when we actually went outside and played softball. She did so great! If I were in her place, I would have been totally frustrated. She, in turn, was amazing and handled herself with determination and grace.

There were days I would go home after work and just sit there thinking of ways to make things more enjoyable for Alex. I remember wishing I could do more and better for her. As a medical professional I knew we were not supposed to take our work home or become so personally attached. I guess I didn't draw the line very well, because I was emotionally connected with Alex and her family. This was one case where I just couldn't help it.

The Alex I knew was very much like any teenage girl. She loved to talk. She even shared dreams about what her wedding would be like and about someday having a family of her own. I would usually just listen, unless I had a specific question. She would politely answer my query and then go right back to talking about the concert she attended or a friend she saw or the event she was planning. I wanted Alex to voice any concerns she had about her condition, but not Alex. If it was on her mind, she didn't show it. For the most part she talked about the future. One would never guess she was facing the ultimate test.

Yes, Alex had a profound impact on my life. She showed me how important it is to live each day to the fullest, yet her message was more than that. We should feel an appreciation for living a normal life. We should have compassion, understanding and acceptance for those who cannot. We should realize that people get sick and struggle to go on. We should embrace them, cherish them and treat them as we would like to be treated. And Alex did one more thing for me. She affirmed my belief in angels, for I know she certainly is one.

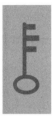

The difference we make in other people's lives is not always visible, not always articulated to us, but it is real.

Harold S. Kushner
Author, *Overcoming Life's Disappointments*

The Porcupine

Friend Talia

Moonlight creeping around the corners of our lawn
When we see the early signs that daylight's fading...

From the song, "Daylight Fading"
Words by Adam F. Duritz
Music by Daniel J. Vickrey, Charles Gillingham & Counting Crows

I close my eyes, and I can still picture my friend Alex and me in elementary school running around the playground chasing boys or playing tag. She had the cutest little raspy voice, and she just loved to have fun and be funny and do crazy things. When I was with Alex I knew I would get dirty and do something out of the ordinary. As we got older, not much really changed, only the people and the places. We obviously matured. Well…a little bit at least!

We would find a way to have fun no matter what we were doing. We knew how to make each other happy. Even when times were rough, we were always there for each other. We could fight and have disagreements too, but it didn't matter. We just "got" each other. She was the sister I never had in my own family, and her parents were my other parents and her brothers were my brothers.

There is no one word to describe Alex. She was just one of those indescribable people. When you were around her, you found yourself feeling happy. And the thing that always stood out for me was her caring nature. She was so selfless. She took care of everything and everyone, no matter what.

I remember a funny little story. One time we were out

driving around, and Alex accidentally ran over a porcupine. Most people would just keep traveling down the road, but not Alex. She turned the car around and went back to see if the animal could be saved. To no one's surprise, the porcupine was dead. Alex couldn't handle the fact that she had killed this poor, innocent creature. It did nothing to deserve its fate, and she insisted on giving it a proper burial before we went on our way. We moved the porcupine to the side of the road, put an old T- shirt and some leaves over it and said some silly little prayer. Nobody else would have done that. It was so sad, yet so hilarious, but so Alex.

There was one other time we were driving around in her little turquoise Plymouth Neon. Her mom had telephoned, and told us that we had to stop by the stationery store, because there was something she had to share with Alex. It turned out to be news about one of Alex's medical tests, and the news wasn't good. We sat there in the parked car, listening to one of our favorite bands, Counting Crows. She took my hand in hers and together we cried. Even now, years later, I cry every time I listen to that song.

After we found out about her cancer, we spent even more time together. I wanted to make sure she knew I appreciated her and loved her. I wanted to make sure she knew how much I cared and that I was going to be there for her every day, all day, whenever she needed me, no matter what.

Alex and I always used to say, "The cancer is just a milestone." We loved using that word to describe the things we were going through. "It's just another milestone."

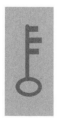

Our task must be to free ourselves...by widening our circle of compassion to embrace all living creatures and the whole of nature and its beauty.

Albert Einstein
German physicist

With Blinders On

Susie

Journal Entry April 30, 1998:

So many people ask, "How are you holding up." I know they mean well.
What must I be made of that they keep asking me? Are they not able to
see how one can be strong, naturally strong at times such as these? It is
only natural to be weak at times, but it seems so natural to be strong.
I guess deep down inside, I am afraid that I could be weak, and that is why
I find it so disturbing.

Bill

Billy and I pretty much had blinders on. As parents we were
going to do everything we could to get our daughter well. We
were going to do everything we could because we are people
who feel, okay, if this doesn't work, you go on to the next thing.
You never give up. There is always something else you can do.

This was one time when we were more in tune with each
other than we had ever been. Over the years we certainly had
our differences. We had different views about a lot of things.
Sometimes it was over the kids, but most of the time over less
important issues. Through it all we shared the same core values
and views about life and about family priorities. As Alex faced
the biggest challenge of her life, we had a clear, common goal,
and that was to get our daughter well. Everything else became
secondary.

If I said, "Billy, I can't take this. I need you to go to the
hospital. I'm too upset." Whatever it was, he responded, "Fine. I'm
there." If he needed me, "Sue, I need you to do this or be there,"

I was. There was never any arguing; nothing was allowed to distract us from the task at hand.

And there were always stories of cancer cases that gave you hope. To share that hope, the hospital staff teamed each patient with a mentor. Alex's mentor was a cancer survivor named Heather. She was a bit older than Alex when she was diagnosed. She was in her 20s and away at college when they found her cancer. She had gone to a 24-hour clinic complaining of leg pain, and the only reason they discovered it was because one of the doctors had seen bone cancer before. Heather had the same cancer as Alex and ended up having 22 chemo treatments and a knee replacement. She was now healthy and doing well.

For me, my emotions on the inside were much different. Sometimes, it felt like I was the person in the famous painting by Edvard Munch titled *The Scream*, but outwardly I couldn't let that show. We had a job to do…a daughter to take care of…a child to keep from falling into depression…to get well.

We moved forward and kept our blinders on.

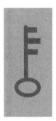

Don't be discouraged. It is often the last key in the bunch that opens the door.

Anonymous

The Hat Fairy

Anonymous

Journal Entry May 2, 1998:

When you returned home for the first time after your amputation, I said to you, "I am the luckiest man in the world to have you as a daughter. You turned around, smiled and said, "Well then, I must be the luckiest girl in the world." You are able to see beauty and life when others would fall apart. What an inspiration!

Dad

You make tradeoffs when you're losing someone to cancer. When the person you love is battling the disease, you hope and pray, "Please save them. Please give me another month and I promise I will take care of people." My father had cancer. In fact he was a survivor of lung cancer. Then seven years into remission he was diagnosed with pancreatic cancer.

The only time I really ever saw my dad cry was the day he lost all his hair from the chemotherapy. He didn't know that I saw him. I had gone over to his house, and he was sitting in the backyard on a lounge chair. His face was all wet from the tears. All of his hair came out in one day. I thought, "How disheartening, to go through all he has gone through and then to lose your hair on top of everything else." It was 23 years ago that my father lost his life to cancer, and that was when I knew I had to do something.

What would be a better gift for someone losing her hair from chemotherapy than a hat? I had always designed great hats, so I decided to make my next hat specifically for a cancer patient.

Once I did, I realized I couldn't stop there. That's how the Hat Fairy came into being. But I didn't want to make hats and just give them to people. I wanted it to be more fun, more magical. My thing is to be anonymous. I want to be the giver, and I want my gift to be both a surprise and uplifting for the receiver. I don't want personal thanks. My reward is in knowing I brought joy to someone at a time when they needed it most. That approach takes some planning, or it won't take much to blow your cover. You have to keep your ears open to find your new secret friend, and you have to find out enough critical information without asking too many questions. That's how I first heard about Alex Graham.

I was at a dinner and overheard a high school student talking about this girl and the great adversity she was dealing with. He talked about how she never stepped back from the challenge. She was always about overcoming cancer and making life happen. My ears perked up and I eased my way into the conversation. I asked, "What is this girl's name? Where does she go to school?" He told me and then I asked, "And what do her parents do for a living?" His answers gave me enough information to get started on my mission, and enough information to begin my new friendship with Alex.

Old vintage hats and decorating hats is a passion of mine. I also have a tie to a children's clothing manufacturing company and access to a knitting machine. Knowing Alex had lost her hair, a cute hat styled for a teenage girl seemed like the perfect gift. Now, making the hat is one thing, but getting it delivered without being revealed is another. I would have to get up in the middle of the night so I could drop off the package on the Grahams' front porch around 3 in the morning. Over the years I'd learned that trying to do that at 11 at night or 5 in the morning made it way too easy to be discovered. It's too common for someone to be coming home late in the evening or leaving early for work.

So I started delivering these surprise packages to Alex's front porch. Sometimes it was a hat, but then it could also be other little things. I tried to bring things that made sense for a young girl like teen magazines, stationery, or a cute T-shirt. Sometimes it would be a gift certificate to a record store or a new book. I would make the timing inconsistent, too. It could be every day for three days and then nothing for a week. What was consistent with each gift was a special note. The message was always a positive affirmation like, "I heard you're doing great" or "Never give up" or "Smile." At the same time, I had to keep my ears open in the community to know how she was doing to make sure the gift and the note were appropriate.

People in town were talking more and more about Alex. I kept hearing inspiring things about her and her determination and positive attitude. Then there came a period when I heard she wasn't doing well, and that she was back in the hospital. I really wanted to know what was going on. Alex and I had never met or ever talked, but over time I had developed my own personal connection with this young girl struggling to beat her cancer. I couldn't seem to get good information, so I decided to call the Grahams' house. The phone rang, but no one answered. I decided to leave a message. It was something like, "I heard Alex was back in the hospital. I just wanted to let her know the Hat Fairy was sitting on her shoulder. I'll leave a note on the porch."

Well, apparently this fairy was not too technologically savvy at the time. A day or so after leaving the message, my phone rang. I picked it up and a voice said, "I know you're the Hat Fairy." I said, "Pardon me? Who is this?" And the woman on the other end of the line replied, "Susie Graham." I said, "I don't know what you are talking about." Susie responded, "Well, we have caller ID." I said, "I am so busted! You are sworn to secrecy!" Susie went on to tell me what a great thing it was for Alex to have the surprise packages and never knowing who was leaving the gifts made it extra fun. She promised not to tell Alex or Bill about our little secret game.

One day I got another call from Susie. She said, "You know, the Hat Fairy was here again, but the Hat Fairy didn't see that Alex left something on the porch for her. It's been there for about 10 days." When I went back there was an envelope taped to the window. Alex left me a card and a letter. She gave me a photograph of her and a picture of her cat. By this time from my notes, Alex knew that I loved animals. In her note, Alex said her fondest wish was that one day I would meet her cat, get to hold it and that she would be able to give me a hug.

Being the anonymous Hat Fairy is what I do. It's been my thing...my way of making a small difference. The truth is, the selfish part of me wanted to run down to the hospital and just hug Alex. I wanted to tell her it would be all right, but I knew if I went to see her I would break down and cry. That's because I know life isn't fair. It's totally not fair, and my crying would not bring comfort to Alex and her family. So, I do my thing, and because of it I feel like I have been blessed a hundred times over.

Alex and I never met and we never talked, but we became close friends. Who would guess that the best gift I have ever received would be a card and note from a teenage girl named Alex?

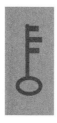

To give without any reward, or any notice, has a special quality of its own.

Anne Morrow Lindbergh
Author and aviation pioneer

Making the Best of a Bad Situation

Friend Sharone

Journal Entry:

I hope my life carries on with one leg even though it's tough now. I have the worst phantom pain ever. It feels like my foot fell asleep, my toe knuckles are scraping on the cement, and my foot is on fire. Other than that, I'm great!

Alex

Alex and I had a turbulent start to our friendship. We went to grade school together, and it was about the fifth grade when Alex discovered what buttons to push that would make me really upset. Girls like to do that to each other at that age. Unfortunately, Alex found it all too amusing. It seemed like every day I would go home and say, "Alex made me cry again today." After numerous calls from my mother to her mother, I think the thrill of the tease wore off, and we settled into a lasting friendship. We lived in the same area, so we ended up playing together on the weekends. We'd climb the birch tree in front of her house and ride our bikes. We did all the things a couple of childhood girlfriends would do.

When we were in the eighth grade we took dance classes together including duet tap. Her brother Robbie would get his karaoke machine out and Alex and I would put these basement talent shows together. For some reason, in every show we would always do a number to Lee Greenwood's "God Bless the U.S.A."

It was funny, because Alex had all these hand signals she would do for all of the parts of the song. She couldn't dance all that well, but she was always quite the performer. Isn't it interesting how some things just stick in your mind forever?

Alex and I went to different high schools, but we remained friends. Naturally we saw less of each other, but we stayed in touch through things like our youth group. Alex had missed a couple of activities. The word was that she was sick and that there was a chance she had cancer. I couldn't really get my arms around it, so I went home and told my parents. Well, Alex had always been a practical joker and loved to pull your leg, so my mom's first reaction was, "Don't think twice about it. She's probably making it all up. She's doing it for her theatrical effect." I was thinking, "Oh, that's sick. What an awful thing to do!" It was at the youth group convention where I found out Alex wasn't joking this time. We were sitting watching some talent acts and she told me as she broke down into tears, "It's for sure cancer." I started crying too. She pulled herself together, and as the night went on she told others and broke down a couple more times. The next day there were no more tears. Alex was saying, "Okay, I'm just going to deal with it. I'm going to fight it, and it will be done and over."

There was never a suggestion of giving up or losing the battle. Through the chemo, the amputation and therapy, everyone remained positive. The doctors remained upbeat. The nurses were upbeat. Her parents were in good spirits, and Alex, well, she was something else. It's like the day of her amputation I went to see her. Instead of complaining about the pain she was experiencing she said, "So, do you want to come in and feel it? Do you want to touch it?" Of course, I was like, "Sure...I guess." She did the same thing to her brother Robbie, and he answered, "I think I'm going to hold off on that, Alex." She teased him again, "No, it's really cool. Touch it!" She made light of it and put others at ease. She always knew how to make the best of a bad situation.

She did things after the amputation that amazed people. One time she was given tickets to watch the Red Wings play for the National Hockey League championship on "Joe Vision" at

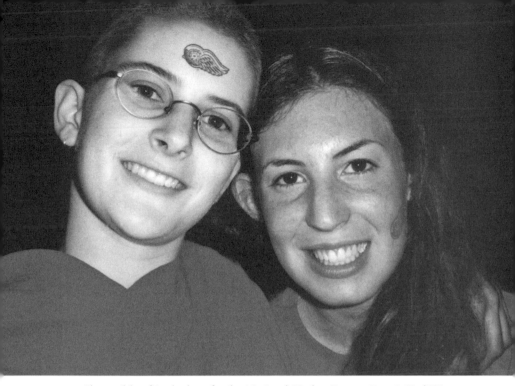

Alex and her friends cheer for the National Hockey League Detroit Red Wings.

Detroit's Joe Louis Arena. There were four of us going, and Alex brought her wheelchair to make it easier for us to get in and around the arena. On the way there, she made sure I didn't get into the car unless I was wearing a team-color red shirt. Once in the car, she whipped out this red mascara and red paint. Suddenly she was putting it all over my hair and writing things on my arm. She was putting it on herself and making all of us put Red Wings tattoos on our faces. By the time we arrived at The Joe, we were awash in red with our hair standing up and sticking out in all different directions. It was a sight to behold.

Once inside the arena, we loaded on one of the elevators, and the doors closed. We had just started to go up, and would you believe it got stuck? We were in this tight space with a whole bunch of other people, and it was really, really hot. There's this one woman who was getting all worked up. She was claustrophobic, and she was scared. She was crying and getting everyone else all upset. Out of nowhere at the top of her lungs Alex started to sing and instructed everyone to sing along. I don't even remember what song it was, but before long all of us had joined in. I was feeling like an idiot, but I was thinking, "Okay, nobody knows who we are."

Finally, Joe Louis security ended up prying the doors open. We were caught between floors, and they shimmied each of us up and out, one at a time, to safety. When we were finally all rescued and standing in the corridor, Alex goes, "I planned that. It's always an adventure with me!" She just had a blast. She loved every second of it. Instead of complaining, she seized the opportunity to turn an inconvenience into a night to remember. Even the woman who was coming unglued ended up laughing and singing.

Alex remedied the situation. She didn't even flinch.

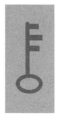

Life is only this place, this time, and these people right here and now.

Vincent Collins
Author, *Acceptance*

Still Time to Laugh

Friend Sarah

Journal Entry May 3, 1998:

You just got out of the hospital. I am so happy to see you able to drive. Finally you have some control over your life. In three days you will be 17. What a fox!

Dad

Alex and I became friends through our synagogue. We were always friendly, but it was when we traveled together to Israel that we became really close. There were about 25 kids on that trip, and we traveled throughout the country on a bus. When you are together 24 hours a day, seven days a week, you form a bond. Four of us girls including Alex really clicked as a group, and we were inseparable from that point on. And Alex…well, it was impossible not to like Alex. She was always doing something that made us laugh. I'd describe her as a troublemaker and an instigator, but not in a negative way. Behind her sometimes zany exterior was the sweetest and most caring person. She was so, so loving. I guess you'd say she was a good troublemaker.

I remember when Alex first told me about her cancer. It's one of those moments that is burned into your memory forever. I was sitting on the carpet in the foyer of our home staring at my reflection in the mirror. I was listening to Alex on the phone as she detailed what had happened at the doctor's. At that point the reality and implications of the diagnosis didn't register. I do remember thinking about a trip we had taken a year earlier. We had gone snow skiing, and on the trip she was complaining that her knee hurt. I can hear her voice saying, "My knee hurts. Rub my knee." We'll never know if she already had the cancer in her body, but that recollection has haunted me to this day.

At 16 years old, I don't think I had any real grasp of what cancer was or what was to come or what Alex was going to face. I didn't understand how her life was going to change, how my life was going to change, how everyone's life around us was going to change. I was too immature to handle it emotionally, so I think I just told myself, "Oh, she has cancer." To me it was like she had a case of the flu. "She'll be fine." I was in denial, and Alex actually helped reinforce my rose-colored view of reality.

She did her best to make sure people didn't feel sorry for her. It seemed as if she purposely made an effort not to talk about her illness, because it started to consume so much of her life. Instead she wanted as much as she could of her normal life. I don't remember her crying. I don't remember her being sad or staying home and moping. To me she was like, "I have cancer, and I'm going to fight it, and I'm going to have my remission party." She always talked about her remission party.

So back to Alex the troublemaker. By this time she had lost her hair, and she had lost her leg. We were out for one of our customary trips about town, and Alex was actually driving her specially equipped Toyota 4Runner. She was wearing her wig, and she hated that damn thing more than anything. It made her head itch like crazy. For the most part, she didn't wear the wig in private or just hanging out with family and friends. Then there were the times when we were out in public. She would wear the wig, because she just didn't want to be stared at.

That night while we were driving, the wig was bothering her so bad that she just ripped it off her head! Well, the timing couldn't have been better. She did it just when there was a lady pulling up in a car next to us. The lady saw her do it, screamed and did a double take. She was even trying to back up her car to see again what had happened. I think she literally thought this girl was pulling out her hair!

We laughed uncontrollably. Alex was cracking up. I was cracking up. We couldn't believe this lady just saw her pull off her wig. Knowing Alex, I think she timed it for the maximum impact. Despite all that she was going through, my dear friend Alex still found a way to laugh.

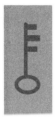

A real friend is one who walks in when the rest of the world walks out.

Walter Winchell
American newspaper and radio commentator

Terrified

Bill

Journal Entry May 11, 1998:

Today I went to lunch at Buggy Works restaurant. When I was leaving the bathroom, I slipped and fell. Ouch! I want my phantom pain to go away. Today I also found out that I have to go to New York with my parents to see the doctor there.

Alex

The cancer traveled in Alex's body, and tumors developed on her lungs. Surgery was required. Beaumont Hospital had pediatric lung surgeons and oncological surgeons on staff, but they did not have a pediatric oncological lung surgeon. We knew Memorial Sloan-Kettering Cancer Center in New York had two of them. Dr. Main was again extremely helpful to us, and on our behalf talked with Dr. Paul Meyers, Chief of Pediatrics at the cancer center. Dr. Meyers agreed to see Alex, so we traveled to New York for an evaluation.

While looking over the X-rays, Dr. Meyer looked at Alex and said, "Alex, do you know you are my most challenging case?" She said, "Yeah." He said, "Do you understand what I'm saying?" And she answered, "Yeah." Arrangements were made for the lung surgery to take place right after Memorial Day weekend and for Susie and me to stay at the nearby Ronald McDonald house.

We returned to the Memorial Sloan-Kettering Cancer Center for the surgery. It was supposed to last about three hours, but the doctor came out to see us in about an hour and a half. He reported, "When I got in there I expected to find less than

20 tumors, but there had to be more than 100. I couldn't take her whole lung out. I had to close her back up." I asked, "Can I give her one of mine?" The surgeon calmly replied, "It's not indicated."

Throughout this ordeal, Susie and I had tried our best to put a positive perspective on the situation, but we also tried to be up front with Alex about what was going on. Now we were faced with a decision of competing values and emotions. Susie and I decided to tell Alex that they didn't get all the tumors. We told her that they got most of them and would try to get the rest with radiation. That was the party line, and we did our best to pull it off.

When the doctor gave us the report, I was so terrified. I was terrified for Alex, and I was terrified for my wife and my boys. I was as terrified as a father could possibly be.

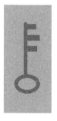

Learning to proceed without a map means taking one step at a time, even though we can't see a clear path to our destination, or even what that destination may be.

Barbara De Angelis, Ph.D.
Author, *How Did I Get Here?*

Save the Children

Bill

Journal Entry June 5, 1998:

I took walking on my own legs for granted, and now I can't do that anymore. Maybe since I helped someone else, I will feel complete...

Alex

Alex went through countless chemotherapy treatments, blood transfusions, loss of hair, dramatic weight loss and a complete hip disarticulation. She handled the pain and discomfort in ways beyond what we imagined possible, but the one thing that drove her and us crazy was the phantom pain. It's called phantom pain because it is a perceived sensation of pain or itching in the limb that was amputated. It can be triggered by changes in the weather, stress or inactivity. Alex would literally ask me to scratch her missing right foot or rub her right leg well after the amputation. She knew it was only phantom pain, but to her and other amputees it is a very real sensation.

One evening, we were sitting at home watching television together. She was trying to keep her mind busy with positive thoughts and off things like the phantom pain. On TV the news reports were telling us of mudslides and devastation in Nicaragua. On came an ad for a Christian Save the Children campaign, and Alex was riveted to the message.

She grabbed the phone, called the 1-800 number and said, "I want to adopt a kid for a year, but listen: I'm 17 years old, and I have cancer, and I'm going to school. I'm real busy. I don't want you calling me every month asking me for more."

She used Susie's and my credit card, but gave us money to pay for the charge. She paid for it from what she made working in her mom's gift and stationery shop. She had always worked at some kind of little job, and even during her battle with cancer she worked when she could. With her leg amputated, no hair and a stocking cap on her head she went about her responsibilities. Still with a smile on her face, she greeted the customers when they entered the store with a cheerful, "Can I help you?"

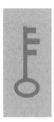

Even if it's a little thing, do something for those who have need of help, something for which you get no pay but the privilege of doing it.

Albert Schweitzer, M.D., OM
Alsatian theologian, musician, philosopher and physician

Alex helps out at her mother's gift and stationery store.

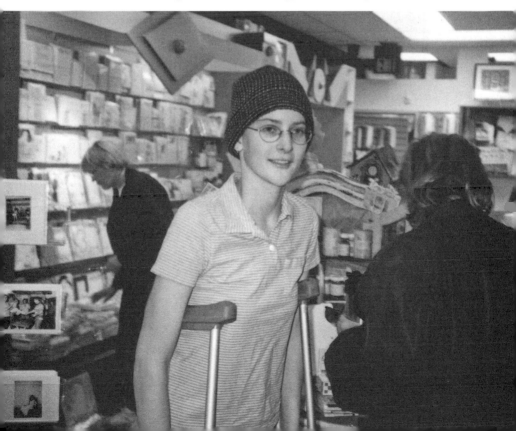

When You're Running Out of Options

Susie

Journal Entry June 9, 1998:

Well, it's Friday, and I came back Monday night from New York. I had the surgery. I guess it went well. The doctor spread my ribs and stretched my muscle, and I woke up with a tube draining out of my chest. We also got some soup at the real "Soup Nazi's" from Seinfeld. I talked to him and he's nice!

Alex

When Bill and I returned with Alex from her lung surgery in New York, we didn't know what to do next. As her parents, we had always kept the blinders on looking for the next best steps we could take to help get our Alex well. We were at Beaumont Hospital to get blood drawn, and I met with Dr. Main. He asked, "Do you want to continue with the chemo? I thought, "What? What do you mean? What does this mean?" We weren't ready to give up, and had anticipated that we would go on fighting the cancer with even stronger chemotherapy. I really didn't expect the doctor's question.

A few days later we heard about a doctor who lived in Australia who had a new protocol for cancer. The theory was that cancer cells cross the maximum number of times a cell can reproduce before dying, known as the Hayflick Limit. The goal is to help the immune system recognize those cancer cells that are not part of the healthy body, so that the immune system will attack them.

The doctor's name was Sam Chachoua. One of his first questions was, "Tell me, was Alex often sick as a child?" I answered, "No! She was never sick." Part of his belief was that some illness in our lives actually can be a good thing. Illness helps build up our immune system, and a strong immune system can help battle other diseases. Because Alex was never sick as a youngster, she didn't have an immune system strong enough to fight off her cancer.

By this time we had clearly run out of options. What Dr. Chachoua offered was an experimental treatment, but we knew we had to do something. We felt what he was telling us made some rational sense. He would make a serum from her blood containing a specific virus. When we told the people at Beaumont what we wanted to do, they were so cool. They said, "We'll work with you on this experimental approach, but only because we do not believe treatment with conventional methods offers any hope of success. We couldn't support this alternative treatment if we felt taking her off chemo was inappropriate." We decided to stop the chemotherapy for 90 days while we tried what we felt to be our only hope. Beaumont took the blood samples we needed, and we kept Dr. Main and his staff informed.

After starting the experimental treatment, Alex actually did better. The doctors at Beaumont were totally surprised. They kept asking, "Alex, are you breathing okay?" She answered, "Oh, yeah. We even went boating and parasailing last week."

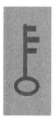

Not knowing when the dawn will come, I open every door.

Emily Dickinson
American poet

Living Life with Gusto

Friends Jessica, Lauren, Sarah, and Tracie

Journal Entry:

I am a feather with the heart of a stallion.

Alex

Life was an adventure for Alex. She was always looking
for something new and different to try. In the summer of 1997 she had traveled out West for a whitewater-rafting trip with an organization called Outward Bound. When the group climbed aboard the raft for the first time, the guide yelled out, "Who wants to be the first one to pilot?" There was a moment of silence as everyone in the raft looked to someone else to respond. Suddenly Alex piped up, "Okay, I'll be the first!" And that was her typical M.O. She was always up for the challenge.

Alex also began making arrangements for an ocean kayaking class and for six months of schooling overseas, but cancer closed the door on those plans. What cancer could not do was squelch her desire to live life with gusto. She found other ways to satisfy her zest for life, even a month after losing her leg. That's when her cousin was getting married. Alex enjoyed a good party, and there she was in the middle of it all. She wore a black dress. She was gaunt, no eyebrows, no eyelashes and wearing her wig, but it didn't stop her from getting out on the floor in her wheelchair to dance. In her own words, she "was doing the swing and having a blast!"

While some plans were put on hold, Alex found other adventures to take their place. For example, she loved the music of the Barenaked Ladies. When they scheduled an appearance in early July of 1998 at a local music store, Alex was determined to be there. She made it clear she was willing to go early the night before and sleep outside if she had to. As part of their new album promotion, BNL was performing a mini-concert at the store, and Alex was not going to miss it. She wasn't shy about what she wanted either. She made sure her wheelchair was right in front of the stage, so she wouldn't miss a thing. She let everyone know there was a "wheelchair coming through" and they should "make way." After the show Alex stood in line for autographs and slipped a note with her name and number to one of the members of the band hoping they would remember her.

That summer she also learned to drive a specially equipped Toyota SUV, went for a hot-air balloon ride, took her friends on jet-ski rides and even went parasailing. But there was one adventure she and I shared that left a lasting impression. My family has always been into riding bicycles. We were heading out to a nearby county park to do some biking, and we invited Alex to come along. We had a tandem bike, and Alex decided she was going to ride it. Keep in mind she had no leg and no prosthetic for this activity, but that wasn't going to stop her. While my parents held the tandem I hopped on the front, Alex maneuvered her thin body up on the rear, and off we went. Needless to say I was apprehensive about what was going to happen. My concerns were quickly set aside. It was almost like she was in better shape than me! Somehow with that one leg she was peddling away and pushing me to keep up!

There just didn't seem to be anything she was afraid of. In fact, it was a bit freaky at times. You actually had to get used to it. You would walk into her house, and you would see the prosthetic leg leaning against the wall. She would rather not wear her wig or a hat. Sometimes we'd go out to dinner. After one bite, she'd have to cover her plate with her napkin, because the sight of food would make her sick. Those were things that sometimes frightened me, and the kinds of images that might cause even the best of friends to shy away. Alex sensed our uneasiness, so she would do what she could to make us feel comfortable. She would take the time to explain things and would do it with a sense of humor and a smile. She would show you her medication port. She would show you her leg and joke about her prosthetic.

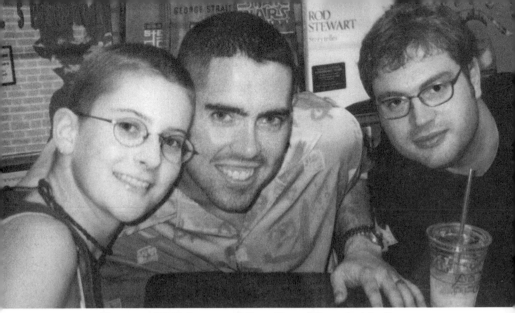

Alex meets Ed Robertson and Steve Page of Barenaked Ladies

You hear stories about people who are faced with a life-threatening illness and end up distanced from their friends. Alex actually gained more friends through it all. She made us look past the bald head and the one leg and see that she was the same person we were friends with all along. Her parents were the same way. The door was always open, and we were always invited and encouraged to come in.

No, there wasn't much Alex seemed afraid of except perhaps losing her friends and missing out on an adventure. Those were things she could influence, and she did. As friends we were welcomed and embraced. As for life, she may have had to change her plans, but she sought out new adventures and made the most of each and every day.

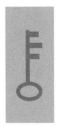

Our purpose in life isn't to arrive at a destination where we find inspiration, just as the purpose to dancing isn't to end up at a particular spot on the floor. The purpose of dancing—and of life—is to enjoy every moment and every step, regardless of where we are and when the music ends.

Wayne W. Dyer, Ph.D.
Author, *Inspiration: Your Ultimate Calling*

Cedar Point

Charles A. Main, M. D.

Journal Entry June 11, 1998:

All my friends leave on Sunday for camp. I really miss school and being able to walk on my own. I really miss freedom, being able to have control of my life. I don't want the cancer to spread, and I can't control that!

I really hope I can go to Cedar Point with the clinic. I'm so excited 4 it!

Alex

Every summer we take a busload of children who are being cared for at the Rose Cancer Treatment Center to the Cedar Point Amusement Park in Sandusky, Ohio. It's one of the things we do for the children to get them away for a day from all the treatments and such. It's a chance for them to do things they might not otherwise get to do. It really gives them something to look forward to, and as the director of Pediatric Hematology and Oncology, it's an event I and the other physicians, nurses and play therapists look forward to as well. We accompany the children as chaperones and medical support. There is about one of us for every two children who are well enough to make the trip.

Now, I've practiced medicine for over 40 years. Someone asked me, "With all the thousands of young patients you've cared for, which ones stand out? I had to answer, "They all stand out." In fact, it's funny. Every once in a while a child I hadn't thought of for a long, long while will pop up in my head. Then, there are certain others I think of quite frequently. Alex is one of those patients.

Alex was a very mature young woman. As far as her medical

care, she was not one to lay back and let the doctors and nurses do whatever they wanted. She asked a lot of questions and wanted to know just what was going on. She was very involved in making decisions about her medical treatment. She always did it in a direct and courteous manner. In working with her it didn't take long to learn that if you were going to do something, you better have sound medical reasoning for doing it. You knew that with Alex, she was going to question you about it.

Often when children have cancer, especially when treatment drags out over time or there are complications, they become angry. Many times they direct that anger at the doctor or other members of the staff. Alex got angry too, but she directed her anger at the situation. She shared her anger and her disappointment, but she was not angry at the medical staff. That's a level of maturity we don't often see in young adults, and a meaningful life lesson for all of us.

One of my all-time, outstanding recollections took place on one of those trips to Cedar Point. Alex was assigned to my group. She and two of the other teenage girls decided to ride on the rollercoaster. The two girls sat in the front seat and Alex was in the back. One of the girls in the front was wearing a wig. As they went over one of the high peaks into a big drop, they all had their hands up in the air. Well, the wig from the girl in the front flew off. She was as bald as could be. As quick as the wig flew off, Alex, sitting in the second seat, caught the wig in mid-air.

Now, there happened to be some boys close in age who had been watching the girls. The three girls were really attractive, so the boys were keeping their eyes on them as they took their rollercoaster ride. They saw this whole thing transpire, and I swear they almost jumped out of the rollercoaster. I mean, it all happened so fast and so clean, that it looked like it was a planned stunt. When the ride stopped, the boys watched as Alex, standing on her one leg, gave the other girl back her wig.

On the bus ride back I happened to sit next to Alex. She was unusually quiet, so I asked her, "Did you have a good time?" And she answered, "Yes, I had a very good time today." She paused for a moment and said, "I think I know what I want for my Make-A-Wish." I said, "What's that, Alex?" She said, "I want to tell people how to treat people that have cancer."

Right away I was thinking that her wish could be a difficult wish to grant. How would you ever do that? So, I thought I would probe a little deeper. I asked, "Why is that your wish?" She answered, "I didn't like the way we were treated, and I didn't like the way people looked at us today."

I guess it was part her age and part her maturity that made her sensitive to those things. She noticed how she had been treated, and because of her caring nature, she was also watching and aware of how others in our group were looked at and treated.

That was a day I will never forget, and the day when Alex's wish took form.

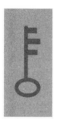

There remain times when one can only endure. One lives on, one doesn't die, and the only thing that one can do is to fill one's mind with the concerns of other people. It doesn't bring immediate peace, but it brings the dawn nearer.

Arthur Christopher Benson
British essayist, poet and author

Returning from Cedar Point

Bill

Journal Entry July 18, 1998:

I got to go to Cedar Point. Yeah!

I have lots of wishes. Wishes about life, about this year and about this month. I wish this nightmare ends soon. I wish the tumors leave and the chemo stops. I wish I did not need a transplant of any sort. Then there is the wish that seems so silly to some, I wish I have hair (enough) for my senior picture. I wish my parents are happy and my brothers and family.

Alex

Susie and I went to pick up Alex when she returned from Cedar Point Amusement Park. We didn't expect to find her mad, but that's what she was.

We had leased a Toyota SUV for Alex, because we wanted her to ride in a very safe vehicle. The thing is, if you have bone cancer and break a bone, the chances are great that the cancer will react by spreading all over. We wanted a vehicle that was stable and not going to slide off into a ditch or anything. So why was she mad?

She informed us that she was mad because we had a nice car, and a lot of the families that she knew with kids in treatment had cars that were blowing oil and everything. "I'm mad too because both of you are here." I said, "Alex, we've both gone to your baseball games. We've both gone to the open houses at school together. We are your parents. Why shouldn't we both be here?" She answered, "Because most of these kids only have one parent here. The other parent has to work or be with the family's other kids."

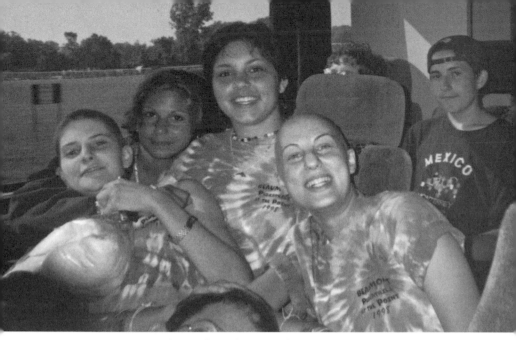

Coming home after a day at Cedar Point Amusement Park.

On the trip she found out that her kind of cancer strikes one out of 125,000 people between the ages of 12 and 25. She also found out she qualified for Make-A-Wish, and she made it clear what her wish was. "I'm going to make a public-service announcement about how to treat kids who have cancer and none of this public-access nonsense. I want it to go on channels 2 and 4 and 7 and everything. I want people to watch it. I want people to learn from it and ask each other, "What do you think?"

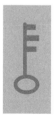

Do all the good you can. By all the means you can. In all the ways you can. In all the places you can. At all the times you can. To all the people you can. As long as ever you can.

John Wesley
Anglican minister and Christian theologian

Head Bobbing

Friend Illana

Journal Entry:

All the time I picture myself with two legs and it's great... but then I look down and cry. I cry so hard. I cry at night and in the car mostly.

Alex

Several of us had signed up to study in Israel for the second semester of our junior year of high school. We had already gone to orientation, and the necessary payments had been made. That was before Alex found out she had cancer. When Alex told me I remember asking, "What's going to happen with our Israel trip?" She said, "Well, I can't go." So right then and there I thought, "I'm not going either." Alex and I did everything together and I couldn't go without her. It wouldn't be any fun.

The summer before our senior year, a bunch of us went to camp together. We had attended the camp every summer growing up. This year we went to participate in what's called a TSF program. It's kind of a junior counselor program. For us it was the pinnacle of going to camp. Being a TSF was a sign you had arrived, and it's like the biggest summer of your life. I was really looking forward to it, but just like studying abroad, I really didn't want to go without my friend Alex.

My parents pushed me to participate anyway. They said, "You're not staying home, and you just can't go to the hospital every day. It's important that you go out and continue to make new friends. We don't want you to miss out. You need to go on with your life too." I did end up going to camp, and I had this horrible feeling of guilt for leaving Alex behind. I know my parents were trying to protect me from being hurt, but it's kind of funny. I was still hurting, because I didn't have my friend with me. Time goes by, but guilt can linger for a long, long time.

That period of time, when I and many of Alex's other friends were at camp, was very difficult for her. She never said anything like, "I'm mad you left" or "I'm depressed because I couldn't go, and you went anyway." I'd call her on the phone and come home now and then to see her. She never said a thing, but I could just tell she was feeling left out and disappointed. A sign to me was when she started to listen to a lot of melancholy, sad music, and that wasn't like Alex at all. The two of us always loved happy music.

Even before she was diagnosed with cancer, we had spent a lot of time driving around in her little Plymouth Neon and listening to fun music. We tried to find songs we could bob our heads to. Everything was fun and happy. She liked the song "Penny Lane" by the Beatles. That was a head bobber. I can still picture us laughing, singing and bobbing our heads. Of course, we both liked the Barenaked Ladies and drove through town, lip-synching the lyrics and smiling all the way down the road.

The lyrics are what I identify with. I listen to music with lyrics that symbolize my mood and state of mind. One night that summer, Alex and I were out driving. This time I was at the wheel and Alex was on the passenger side. We had just arrived at my house and as I was pulling the car into my parent's garage, the song "Wind Beneath My Wings" came on the radio. I turned off the engine and looked at Alex and said, "This song makes me think of you." We just sat there silently, staring into the darkness while listening and feeling the words and Bette Midler's voice touch our hearts. Believe it or not, it was one of the very few serious moments Alex and I had shared throughout her illness. Little did we know that not far down life's road, Alex would be touching the hearts of millions through that very song.

A loving silence often has far more power to heal and to connect than the most well-intentioned words.

Rachel Naomi Remen, M.D.
Author, *Kitchen Table Wisdom*

The Wish

Susan Lerch, Make-A-Wish Foundation

Wish Application, September 2, 1998:

I want a commercial to raise money for cancer funds, for people who can't afford the medication. I want to have me and some other patients from the Rose Cancer Center in it telling people not to take things for granted. I want it to tell people not to laugh at us because we don't have hair. It's not my fault I lost my leg to cancer. My friend Julie has a tumor on her voice box. She squeaks when she talks, and people laugh.

I want to tell people that all these kids have been through so many shots, chemos, hair loss and bone marrow transplants. How bad could everyone else's lives be compared to us? So, don't take things for granted, especially because we miss out on lots of stuff that our friends get to do.

I also want "Wind Beneath My Wings" to play in the background. And can my commercial be on a famous TV station and be national?

Alex Graham

I've been with the Make-A-Wish Foundation of Michigan for over 10 years. Initially I was hired as the Executive Director. In 1998 we were granting in the range of 125 to 200 wishes a year to Michigan residents. Because of the caring and generous support in our state we granted our 5,000th wish in 2007.

About 75 percent of those wishes involved some kind of destination wish such as a trip to Disney World. Yes, it's the wish of most children to go to Disney World, but in these cases, it's much more than just a trip to a fun location. It's a time for the child and her or his family to have something to look forward to, to have no worries for a few weeks, for everybody to be kind and loving and generous. The wish becomes something the family can focus on, so they can have this one worry-free period of time that is all positive. It doesn't eliminate the pain or take it away, but it can help the child and her family by just knowing other people cared.

Many people believe Make-A-Wish has this magic wand, and that everyone just gives us everything to make any wish happen. It's true that there are many generous and giving individuals and businesses, but it also takes a lot of volunteers and cash to make each wish become a reality. Sometimes there is also a misconception that a child's illness must be considered terminal in order to be eligible for Make-A-Wish or that a wish is based on a family's financial needs. Those conditions are not true at all. In fact, many of our kids become survivors. When they become adults, many become huge supporters of the wish experience. While we do have to practice what we call "wishful management," it is our goal never to turn away an eligible child. In the end, the thing I love about what we do as an organization is that we are true advocates for children and families. People, many of whom are strangers, come together with love, generosity and compassion to support a child and family in distress.

When Alex's wish came in my reaction was, "Wow! This is interesting. It was so different from the majority of wishes that came across our desk. How are we going to do this one?" My reaction is always, "Never say never." I draw on all the old adages like "Where there's a will there's a way." When I read this particular request, I was thinking, "This one is unique and incredible." I wanted to go and meet this girl and find out a bit more about what she was thinking and what was actually feasible. How do we create this "commercial," as she described it, and do so in a way that it will carry her message? How do we really put it all together? How do we go about getting permission to use something like Bette Midler's "Wind Beneath My Wings"? When it's done, how do we actually get airtime? The wish was such a selfless request, and those come along once in a blue moon. That doesn't mean other wishes aren't incredibly important and don't foster a sense of community, but Alex's wish was truly extraordinary.

We had worked in conjunction with a wonderful program called The Partnership for Humanity. Sponsored by the Detroit Newspapers, the program links advertising agencies with nonprofit organizations to create awareness ads that run in *The Detroit News* and *Detroit Free Press* over the course of a year. We were looking for a way to increase the visibility and understanding of our organization in the community, and The Partnership for Humanity connected us with BERLINE, an advertising, public relations and communications agency. About that time, Jim Berline became a member of our board. When I approached Jim with Alex's wish, there was no hesitation on his part. It was through him and his agency that we had a chance to make this one-of-a-kind wish for a "commercial" come true.

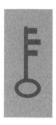

That is the essence of what it is to be human...to be kind and compassionate to one another.

Susan Lerch, President and CEO
Make-A-Wish Foundation of Michigan

Making the Wish a Reality

Jim Berline, Chairman, BERLINE

Journal Entry:

It's been so frustrating lately. First my leg is so big and goofy. Second, I walk like an inchworm. And third, I'm scared to go to school for just one class. I don't know why, but I am.

Alex

After 10 years as an advertising executive, I decided to start my own agency. So, 24 years ago Berline was formed. I always felt companies had a responsibility to give back to the community, and one of the ways my company could do that was by providing select charities with agency services. We focused a majority of those efforts on child-oriented charities. In 1998 we completed a video for a children's charity called Variety. The video ended up winning a special recognition, and I was attending a luncheon to receive the award. There were a number of people at the luncheon representing various not-for-profit organizations. There I met a woman who was a developmental planner for The Make-A-Wish Foundation. We got to talking about the great work that Make-A-Wish does, and she shared with me that one of their biggest challenges was in marketing and communications. I said, "My agency can solve that problem." That's when Berline started providing pro-bono agency services to Make-A-Wish.

Not long after that, I was invited to serve on the board for the Make-A-Wish Foundation of Michigan. I was only on the board about a month when its president came to me and said,

"Jim, I got this wish, and I don't know just what to do with it." She handed me a handwritten wish from an Alex Graham and said, "This young girl has a very ambitious dream." I read the note and said, "Not a problem. We can grant this wish right now."

The next step was to hold a series of meetings with Alex, her parents and the president of Make-A-Wish. In those discussions I learned about Alex, about her condition, and about her trip to Cedar Point. I learned more about her wish to tell other people that it wasn't their fault she and her friends had cancer and that they just wanted people to smile at them. By this time Alex's leg had already been amputated, and because she was going through treatments, she had major ups and downs. She would get spurts of energy where she could meet with us and then there would be times when she would be in bed. So it depended on where she was with her treatments as to whether we talked on the phone or whether we would meet in person.

We talked with Alex at length about what she wanted to accomplish with her TV spot. We wanted it to be a reflection of how Alex felt, and we wanted it to be as much in her words as possible. Based on her input we would draft copy and take it to Alex. She would say, "I wouldn't really say it that way. I would say it this way. This is more my words." We took her input and prepared a revised script. When she read it she said, "That's what I want to say, and I want the music to be 'Wind Beneath My Wings' by Bette Midler." Now, if you asked most celebrities to let us use their hit recording for no cost they would say, "You're crazy" or they would give you limited rights with some kind of hook attached. But we got in touch with Bette Midler, and she was remarkable. She said, "You got it. You've got the song and my voice."

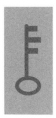

Dream no small dreams for they have no power to move the hearts of men.

Johann Wolfgang von Goethe
German writer and poet

When One Door Closes

The Shoot

Jim Berline

When a child gets cancer, the whole family gets cancer.

Bill Graham

Alex spent a lot of time selecting the people she wanted to be in her "commercial." She wanted to include specific kids she got to know while going through treatment at the hospital. The next step was for me and other members of the Berline agency team to meet with the children and make sure their parents had an understanding of what was involved in producing a television spot. We knew that if we were going to bring all these kids who were in various stages of their illness and treatment to the studio at the same time...well, it was going to be a very long and demanding day. We didn't want anyone mad or disappointed because of the tiring process. We also needed to know how each of the children felt during the course of a typical day, so that if they tended to feel better between, say 8 and 10 in the morning, we could try to get them on camera in that period. Finally, we worked our way through all of the pre-production planning, and the shoot was scheduled.

On the day of the shoot all of the kids showed up. The parents brought cameras, because they were trying to capture every moment with their child that they could. And, typical of a Make-A-Wish experience, other family members were participating as well. Make-A-Wish is not just an individual gift. It is something meant for the entire family. While this was Alex's wish, the brothers and sisters of all the kids involved were there

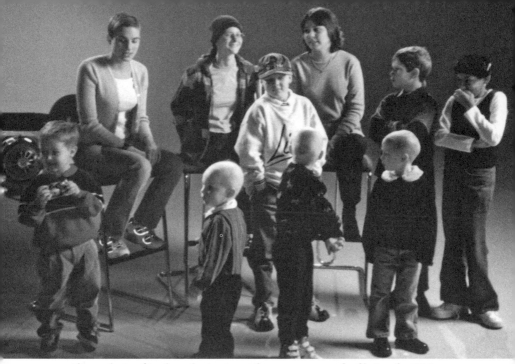

Alex and nine friends under treatment for cancer prepare for filming the PSA.

watching, listening and sharing in the day. Some of the kids were just plain wired, because they were so excited. This was an "on" day for them. They were running around. For others, it was a "not so good" day. They were carried in. Some were sleeping. Some were wearing stocking caps. Some were nothing but smiles from the time they arrived and others were crying. There were a lot of emotions at play.

To see and work with these children, each of whom knew they had a life-threatening disease, was remarkable, and to watch their parents interact with them was a life-changing experience for everyone on the project. To begin with, the Detroit production film and video community had rallied around the wish. These were some of the best professionals and facilities in the business, yet the director, assistant director, cameraman, crew and studio were all donated. I think the only thing we ended up paying for was the film stock, and even that was discounted.

Everyone's heart was touched by the experience. For

example, one of the crew members wanted to personally pay for everyone's lunch. He said, "No, we aren't asking anyone to pay today. I'm going to write a check to the caterer to feed these families. I'm going to pay because of what this means to me." That crew member didn't come to the shoot with the intention of buying meals for 30 to 40 people, but once engaged in the significance of what was happening, it took him less than a second to make the decision to do so.

Alex was engaged in every aspect of the day, too. She wasn't demanding, but she made the studio production very much her deal. She orchestrated her vision in a very specific and positive way. She would say things like, "Come on over and stand here," and "I want you over here by me." As far as set design and treatment, it became an easy creative decision to go with a black-and-white approach. Then, because of the nature of the message, it also made sense not to go for those perfectly framed commercial-like shots. That look wasn't this message. Instead we wanted the audience to feel the day-to-day reality faced by these young cancer patients. When the one little girl spontaneously offered, "Too many pokes," the simplicity and honesty of her words captured the reality of it all. That phrase wasn't in the script Alex had originally written and approved, but we all agreed the words of the little patient's with cancer belonged.

Everyone's time and all the facilities were donated that day, yet everyone was compensated in a far more meaningful and lasting way.

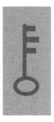

Human greatness does not lie in wealth or power, but in character and goodness. Give whatever you have to give. You can always give something, even if it is a simple act of kindness.

Anne Frank
Author, *Stories and Events from the Annex*

BNL

Bill

Journal Entry October 19, 1998:

You will not believe what happened to me last week. Wednesday night I got a call from Ed Robertson of the Barenaked Ladies. I almost died. He asked me how far the Palace was from Beaumont Hospital. He said he might visit me. Then on Thursday he showed up with a bouquet of flowers, three T-shirts, stickers and a poster, and a guitar. We talked. He sang five songs. It was the best thing in the world and the sweetest thing that anyone's ever done for me. The next day I was in the paper and on the radio and on the Internet. WOW. I just love him. What a great guy. I'm just so amazed. What a rush.

Alex

In the summer of 1997 I had attended a Northwest Airlines charity auction, and at the auction I won tickets to the next year's MTV Music Awards. Knowing how my daughter, Alex, loved music, I knew going to the awards would be special for her and a memory maker for a father and daughter. The package included travel, lodging and a limo ride to and from the awards. When Northwest Airlines contacted us about flight arrangements to Los Angeles, I explained Alex's health issues and asked if I could pay to upgrade the flight to first class. That way Alex wouldn't have to hobble to the seats back in coach. Northwest happened to be in the middle of a strike at the time, but when they heard about Alex, they not only arranged for us to fly on another carrier, they gave us four first-class seats so that Susie and I and a friend of Alex could accompany her on the trip. Northwest Airlines was wonderful!

In Los Angeles, they booked our stay at a hotel used by many of the people in the music industry. We were outside in the courtyard of the hotel having breakfast, and over the loud speaker we heard, "Paging Billy Ray Cyrus. Paging Billy Ray Cyrus." That's when we realized he was sitting at the table next to us. Alex was thrilled by it all, and caught glimpses of other singers and musicians. Later that evening, we rode to the theater like rock stars in our limo, and thoroughly enjoyed the awards show.

But that wasn't Alex's biggest thrill at the awards. Susie, Alex, Alex's girlfriend and I were walking out of the auditorium and Alex shouted, "There's Ed!" Just 20 feet away stood Ed Robertson of the Barenaked Ladies. Ed spotted Alex and walked over to say "hello." He talked with her for a bit and even gave her and her friend the BNL e-mail address. Alex was blown away and was looking forward to seeing him in concert in Detroit on October 17.

Alex's excitement from the MTV awards turned into disappointment. October was a very difficult month. Her blood counts dropped so much that within a one-week span she was in Beaumont Hospital for three transfusions. In her journal she wrote, "I'm losing my hair again, so I tried to bleach it. I still have one leg and a lot of phantom pain. I haven't been able to wear my prosthetic in a few weeks because I am so weak and the chemo knocked me out and I'm just hurting. I'm going in again for chemo and I'll be missing the BNL concert again."

The day before the Barenaked Ladies were to appear at the Palace of Auburn Hills just outside of Detroit, Alex got a phone call from Ed Robertson saying he was in Cleveland and he was going to try to call her when he got to Detroit. Apparently Alex's friend made good use of that e-mail address Ed gave them at the MTV awards. She filled him in on how he could get in touch with her. That evening when I got home from spending time with Alex at the hospital, the phone rang. The caller ID read "GUND." I knew it must be from the Gund Arena in Cleveland. I figured it had to be Ed, and it was. I explained Alex's condition and prognosis. Ed said he didn't realize that Alex had lost her leg to cancer. He thought maybe she had been in a car accident. He wanted to know what her favorite flowers were, and he said, "I'm going to try to come by."

I remember the day. Susie was at the hospital, and I had gone to buy her a latte at the local Starbucks. I told the clerk that it looked like Ed Robertson of BNL was going to be visiting my daughter. She said, "I can't believe it! Their limo driver was just here and he said he had just dropped Ed Robertson off at Beaumont to see some patient." Ed had kept his promise and at that very moment was visiting Alex.

Ed walked into Alex's room and said, "You can't go to the concert, so the concert is coming to you!" He had his guitar, and it was as Alex wrote in her journal, Ed performed five songs just for her. Apparently Ed hadn't told anyone exactly where he was going. Alex was super- impressed by the fact that Ed had cancelled media interviews because he "needed to visit his friend."

Alex wasn't the only one who was impressed. By the time I got back to the hospital, Ed had already left. After Alex shared the details of his visit, I immediately called a friend who was a music critic to fill him in on what had just transpired. The next morning an article appeared in the paper, and before we knew it, the story was reported in newspapers and on radio stations across the country. Casey Kasem even picked up on it, and whenever he played a BNL song on his radio show he shared the story about Ed visiting Alex. When Ed heard about the media coverage he sent an e-mail to Alex saying, "I'm sorry. I don't know how that got out to the press." Alex responded, "Well, that's my dad and his big mouth."

Ed contacted her again before a BNL concert scheduled for December in Grand Rapids. His e-mail said, "Alex, can you make it to the concert? If you can, I'll leave four tickets for you." Alex wasn't doing well, but she insisted she was doing well enough to make a trip to see the Barenaked Ladies. About 3 o'clock in the afternoon on the day of the concert the phone rang. Susie answered it and said, "Alex, it's for you." As Susie handed over the phone she mouthed, "I think it's Ed." It was, and as soon as Alex hung up, she, three of her friends, Susie and I got in the car and headed for the west side of the state. Alex got there in time

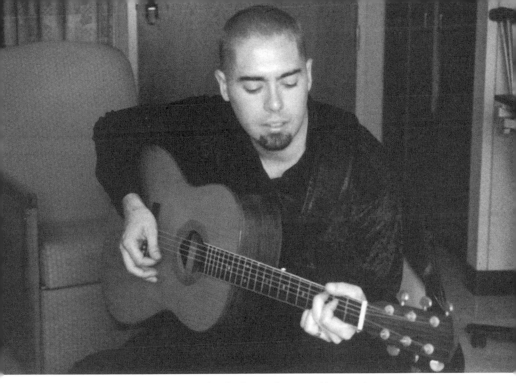

Ed Robertson stops by the hospital to give Alex a private concert.

to see Ed and her favorite group in person one more time.

That month, *Rolling Stone* magazine carried an article written by Will Hermes about the Barenaked Ladies. In it he wrote, "At the end of the day, perhaps this is what Barenaked Ladies are all about: the ability to make life's load a little lighter." He was writing about the group's music and humor, but to us, his words meant so much more. For us, Ed Robertson reached out and made a difference. When cancer was closing doors, Ed made life's load a little lighter for a teenage girl named Alex.

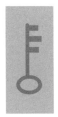

The doors we open and close each day decide the lives we live.

Flora Whittemore
Author

Searching for Comfort and Strength

Susie

Journal Entry December 22, 1998:

Grandpa, it has been one whole year since I got sick. How much longer will I go through this? Hopefully I will have hair by my birthday, or even yours would be great. Maybe you can put in a good word for me up there. But not too good, because I don't want to end up there now. I still have a whole life to live.

Alex

The thing about Billy and me is that we are creative people. As Alex's parents, our mindset was, "Okay, if this doesn't work, we'll move on and we'll try this." We had the best doctors, we sought out second opinions and we had a lot of contacts in the medical community. We had all these good people on our side, and they were telling us that we were doing everything right. It's funny, because as husband and wife, we find ourselves disagreeing a lot. We share core values, but more often than not, we are totally different in our opinions and attitudes. But, when it came to our daughter, Alex, we were like a well-oiled machine. We were completely in sync, and I drew a lot of strength from that. For so many couples, having a child with medical or other problems pulls them apart. In our case it was never like that. We shared a common goal, and that was to get her well.

When your child is undergoing treatment for cancer, you spend a lot of time sitting and waiting, so I did a lot of reading. Some of what I read was very uplifting. I read Bernie Siegel's

Love, Medicine & Miracles. I read *Kitchen Table Wisdom* by Rachel Naomi Remen, M.D., who wrote about people who had some kind of serious illness. The stories tell about how they recovered or how they went through their ordeal and emerged with some kind of positive feeling or life-changing experience. I was touched and strengthened by Mitch Albom's *Tuesdays with Morrie*, and I read several of Harold Kushner's works including *When Bad Things Happen to Good People*. His writings are phenomenal, and strongly influenced the direction of my thinking.

Did I pray? Yes, but it was hard. I wondered, "How can I pray my daughter gets well when this floor is filled with children suffering... struggling to survive?" You know, if I'm going to pray, I'm going to pray for everyone. You know, like, "God, please make my daughter get well." Well....Why? Why make my daughter well and not make the other child in the other bed well? What about this child and that child? What about that family? Why would God make my daughter well but not make their son or daughter well? So, those are just some of the philosophical and emotional issues I wrestled with.

My faith changed and I changed. My whole world was turned upside down. I mean, when I was growing up and I wanted something, say, like a violin, I prayed for something and unfortunately, in my case, I got it. Now, I really had to realign what I felt and what I believed. My beliefs have come to align more with Harold Kushner's thoughts. There are things that happen randomly, that we have no control over. This actually became a very, very comforting belief for me.

I have a very strong belief in God, but I also believe there is a randomness in life. That says to me you didn't do something three years ago that God is punishing you for now. I remember reading the book *Cold Sassy Tree* by Olive Ann Burns in which a 12-year-old boy who got caught on a railroad track but somehow managed to survive. In the story he questioned why God let him live. His grandfather answers the boy with a question of his own. "Still and all, common sense tells you this much; everwhat makes a wheel run over a track will make it run over a boy if'n he's in the way. If'n you'd a-got kilt, it'd mean you jest didn't move fast enough, like a rabbit that gits caught by a hound dog. You think God favors the dog over the rabbit, son?"

I remember the cantor from our synagogue would come at night, bring his guitar and play songs for Alex. I asked him about the fairness of life and he said, "Susie, you know, sometimes, for some things, there just are no answers." And you know, there again, that is the answer.

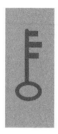

People who pray for miracles usually don't get miracles...
But people who pray for courage, for strength to bear the unbearable, for the grace to remember what they have left instead of what they have lost, very often find their prayers answered.

Harold S. Kushner
Author, *When Bad Things Happen to Good People*

Observations of a Primary Nurse

Nurse Sue

Journal Entry

I'm so glad I have family and friends who love me so much. I never want to lose that feeling. Right now I'm crying and I don't know if it's because I'm tired or if I'm mad or if I'm sad from the flick I just saw. I guess it's the whole world that's hurting me now.

Alex

I had been on maternity leave with my youngest son, and was just returning to work at the hospital. I was one of the nurses assigned to work with adolescents who had some form of cancer. The first thing I heard about was this certain patient and her family and friends. They were causing a stir. The other nurses said they couldn't believe how ambitious this young girl was and how she wasn't letting her diagnosis stop her. The patient turned out to be Alex.

In most cases, children are usually diagnosed in the hospital. First they go to surgery, and from that there is a pathology report. Then additional tests are run to see if the cancer has spread. That process takes about three to five days. Based on that information, a team discusses the case and what type of treatment plan should be followed. The treatment plan is called the protocol. Protocols for osteogenic sarcomas, like Alex's, usually cover a period of nine months to a year.

Typically, every one to three weeks, a child on this protocol would come to the hospital for chemotherapy and a four-to five-day stay. That doesn't count the times when the patient's blood count goes too low and they get a fever. In between all of this, the child usually comes to Beaumont's Rose Cancer Center at least two times a week for blood counts, a possible exam and dressing changes.

In 1998 at the time Alex was in the hospital, we had what were called primary and secondary nurses. If one of those nurses was on duty, she had precedence to take care of her assigned patients. So even if you were assigned to a different hallway, if your patient was in, you got to go over and help care for them. Since a lot of the nurses were on 12-hour shifts, it meant that each patient typically dealt with only two to three nurses.

Working with patients as a primary or secondary nurse, you can't help but develop relationships with the children and their families. There are certain ones, too, who just seem to grab your heart strings. My mom used to say to me, "You cannot take care of these children like you do. You become too attached. Their situations are breaking your heart." You know, sometimes your heart is broken, but that is overshadowed by a feeling of being blessed. People can say "thank you" to us, but what we do is our job. That's what we are here for. The way I look at it, the children have been brought to us to teach us something. That's exactly what Alex did for me.

The first thing I noticed about Alex was her attitude. She may have been bald and she may have been pale and she may have lost a lot of weight, but the spunk she showed was inspirational. You never really saw her in a slump, and that is uncommon for kids her age. Teens start to lose their identity. They are faced with not being able to go to certain things at school, and if they go to school at all, they can't always participate. Some end up being home-schooled in addition to being out of the mainstream while going through treatments. It doesn't take much for them to become isolated. The separation gets to the point where some don't even want to go back to school. Alex couldn't wait for her treatment to be over, because she was anxious to get back to life as it was and move on with big plans for the future.

Unbelievable support was the second thing I saw, especially from Alex's friends. It was almost as if they were admitted into the hospital with her. As soon as she was checked in her room, they began showing up after school and between their activities. They were awesome, and their dedication to their friend never wavered. They would come to watch a movie with Alex or to play music or to talk about their plans. They would spend time together and act just like they were hanging out together at home. I think Alex was their inspiration, and they were hers. Fortunately, Alex's parents and the parents of her friends encouraged them to stay involved. Some parents actually discourage visitors, and some friends shy away out of fear or because they are self absorbed. That was not the case here. Alex's parents, brothers, friends and family provided her with a sense of normalcy at a time when she really had less and less control.

The third thing I observed was Alex's concern for others and a desire to give back. You know, working in a hospital I see a lot of people who get bitter for every reason you can imagine. They are often angry or sad and depressed. Then I see a group who try to cope with their situation and do the best they can. On rare occasions I see individuals and families who take on the struggle and grow from tragedy. Even though the experience is heartbreaking, it changes their lives and, because of it, they want to change the lives of others in a positive way. Alex had her little attitudes from time to time, but more often than not, her first concern was for others. She loved her friends and family and tried not to burden them with her condition. She talked to and cared for other children on the floor. She knew the emotional pain the other children felt when they were looked at differently, and she involved them in sharing her message to the world.

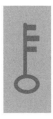

It is the intuitive wisdom of the heart that can help us on our journey of discovering new doorways.

Barbara De Angelis, Ph.D.
Author, *How Did I Get Here?*

Our Last Talk Was a Fight

Friend Jason

Journal Entry January, 1999:

Pain. It's a funny thing. It can hurt you in so many ways.

Alex

We were no longer dating, but Alex and I remained close. My buddy and I went to visit her in the hospital when she was going to have her leg amputated. She had told me on the phone how much she hated what was about to happen, yet when we visited, I couldn't believe how she was handling it. I could not believe this girl's spirit. She was so positive and even joking with the doctor.

From that point on I finally realized how bad this all was turning out. I couldn't believe that for the rest of her life she would only have one leg. I couldn't believe seeing her in a wheelchair.

Part of me was so mad. This was not supposed to happen. In some ways, this just wasn't Alex anymore. She had no hair and one leg. She was getting thinner all the time, and the medicine was causing mood swings. The other part of me was totally amazed. She went on with her life and was enthused about the future. She used her wheelchair or her prosthetic or her crutches to get around. She even invited me to go to a concert in Grand Rapids to see the Barenaked Ladies. I mean, I was a college student worrying about things like getting through my classes, and here was this girl battling cancer. She had one leg amputated, yet she is going to concerts and worrying about getting good seats. I didn't know exactly what to think or do. I was angry about the whole situation, but I was blown away by her positive attitude and her will to go on.

I called her frequently from my college dorm room. I mean, she was still my best friend. We would talk about everything and have these little fights about friendship things. I'd tell her something about what I had done or she would hear things through the grapevine. She'd say, "You didn't tell me about that before" or "Why did you go out with that girl and not tell me?" For a period of time she sounded the same, but then I noticed she was coughing a lot. Every time we talked she seemed to be coughing more and more. I said to her, "Seems like you have a bad cough." She answered, "Yeah, I'm coughing a lot and having more trouble breathing. I'm having trouble catching my breath." I was thinking, "Oh, my God. Maybe I was wrong and she's not going to beat this thing."

It had been quite some time since we agreed not to be girlfriend and boyfriend, yet I still thought she had feelings for me. I know I still had feelings for Alex. Then in December I went to this party. I spotted this cute girl, and before long we were talking. I ended up getting her phone number and calling her the next day. We made plans to go together to another party on New Year's. The day after making those plans, Alex called and asked, "Do you want to hang out for New Year's?" I stumbled, "Uh… no, I can't." She quizzed, "Why not?" I'm like, "Oh, I'm just going to a friend's house."

After New Year's, I gave Alex a call. We hadn't talked in a couple of days, and I could tell she was acting different toward me. I asked, "Are you mad at me or something?" There was what seemed like a very long silence, then she answered, "You know, it's just because I don't feel good. I'm sick."

"No, there's something else wrong." There was another long pause. Suddenly she started yelling at me. "Why didn't you tell me about this girl? Why did I have to find out from someone else? You're not the good friend you pretend to be!"

"I am your best friend. You know I still care about you so much. You know that I love you, but there's nothing I can do about that now. There's nothing I can do about this whole thing. This is just the way it is. It's not that I don't want it to be different. It's not that I don't want to tell you everything, but you're sick right now."

"I'm not mad because I like you or anything. I'm mad because if you were my best friend you would tell me about these things. I just don't believe you anymore. You don't really care. How can you be my best friend and not tell me what's going on?"

Alex kept hanging up on me, and I kept calling back, trying to talk to her...trying to make sense of it all. She kept coughing and coughing. I said, "It doesn't sound like you are doing too well right now. She's like, "I'm fine. I'm fine." The conversation kept going in circles, and it wasn't going anywhere good. Eventually we said goodbye.

The next day, I got a call from one of Alex's close friends who said, "They took Alex to the hospital, and it doesn't look good. She had to be put on a breathing machine."

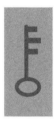

Perhaps the most delightful friendships are those in which there is much agreement, much disputation, and yet more personal liking.

George Eliot
English novelist

Try a Smile

Jim Berline

I didn't know the power of a wish. I thought Alex's wish was just going to be her wish. I had no idea how it would affect so many people.

Bill

The studio shoot of Alex's wish was a long and emotional day, but it was also a personally rewarding day for me and everyone working on the project.

The next step in the process of producing a television spot is the post-production phase. First the film is sent off for processing, and then it is prepared and organized for the editing process. We were all ready to move forward, but we had to wait until Alex was strong enough to meet us at the editing session. When she was finally able to come in we started to fit things together. We got pretty far into it, and Alex just ran out of gas. It was enough for that day, and she went home. We had the script and knew the direction, so we kept going until the picture edit was pretty much complete.

We were at the point where the picture and the music were to be put together. Alex really wanted to be a part of that, but we weren't sure when she would call back and be well enough to join us. My instincts were to keep going. I instructed the Berline team to do so and told them, "If she calls back and is able to participate, we can always work with that. If she doesn't, the commercial will be that much closer to completion and fulfilling her wish."

One day I was down at the Detroit Athletic Club playing

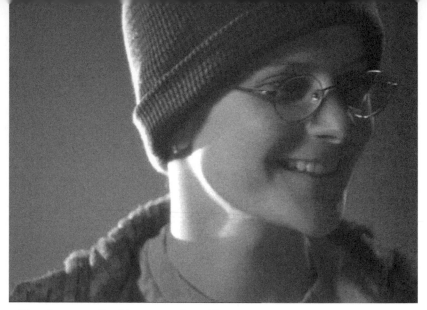

Alex shares a smile of her own as her wish to promote cancer awareness comes true.

in a squash tournament. I had a match at 10 a.m. and another scheduled for 3 p.m. Normally I stay there between matches. For whatever reason, this day I went home and my message light was flashing. I checked it, and it was from Alex's aunt. In it she said, "Jim, we just wanted to see where you were in the commercial because Alex is at Beaumont, and we have some bad news. It looks like she may not make it the next 36 hours, and she wants to see her commercial." Ironically, we had just finished the commercial the day before.

I immediately called the Graham house and there was no answer. Then I called the phone in Alex's room and there was no answer. Finally I called Beaumont and got connected to the nurse in the pediatric cancer ward. I asked, "Is Alex there?"

The nurse said, "Yes."

"Can I talk to Sue or Bill?"

"They are talking to the doctor right now."

"Oh…well I need to talk to them, so whoever gets this message first, please have them call me right back."

Shortly after, Susie called me back. I said, "Susie, I finished the commercial. I've got it. What is the status with Alex? I will be there in 30 minutes. Is there a place for her to see it?

Sue said there was a TV with built-in VCR, so I took off for the Berline offices, picked up the video and drove over to Beaumont as fast as I could. I went to the nurses' station and said, "Here. I need to get this video to Alex. She is expecting it."

The nurse said, "No, you are taking it down to her room. We aren't taking it down. She wants you to bring it."

I wasn't expecting this. I walked down the hall and looked in the room. There she was. I hadn't seen her for quite some time. Now she looked to be half the size she had been, and she had on an oxygen mask. I looked at her and thought, "Holy Jesus! I don't know how I'm going to deal with this."

Susie and Bill were there. I went in. Alex couldn't talk. I leaned over and gave her a kiss on her head and said, "I think you are going to like this." I could tell that little kiss hurt. She was so tender that it actually left a slight impression.

We put the cassette in the VCR. Alex wanted to press the play button on the remote. She hit it. We heard Bette Midler start singing and Alex saw herself on the screen. I started to cry. Susie was crying. Bill was crying. Alex couldn't cry aloud, but tears were coming out of her eyes.

All of us just sat there in silence for what seemed like days, but it was probably only five minutes. Then I asked, "Would you like to see it again?" So we played it again. I said, "Well, I better go now." I went over to give her another little kiss, and she said, "Perfect." That's all she said: "Perfect."

Bill walked me to the elevator and told me, "That commercial is what she has been waiting for, and it's an amazing piece."

I said, "All I want you to do is to call me when whatever happens, happens."

I went to the hospital parking lot, got in my car and just sat there for a moment. I've got three kids, so I decided to call each one of them. I said, "I am going to talk to you like you have never heard me talk to you. So just don't think I am drunk, and don't be mad at me. I just need you to know how much I love you and how much you mean to me."

The next morning I was expecting to have a phone call from the hospital, but I heard nothing. I called the nurses' station at Beaumont and the nurse said, "Alex is still with us. She has shown the commercial to her friends and all the kids in the hall. She wants to show it to her rabbi."

Later that day, I got the call from Bill.

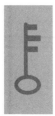

Did you ever know that you're my hero,
and everything I would like to be?
I can fly higher than an eagle,
'cause you are the wind beneath my wings.

Excerpt from "Wind Beneath My Wings"
Words by Larry Henley and Jeff Sibar

Let Ed Know

Bill

Journal Entry

In the morning when the sun will rise protect me from bitterness, evil and lies. Oh God, be the source of all my healing and stop this pain and suffering which I'm feeling. Give me strength and courage in my time of need... Redeem my body and soul from this plague. It's been enough... Oh Merciful One, remind me you are with me. I shall not fear, but as of now there's no direction to steer. All I ask is for an end to all this grieving.

Excerpt from Alex's Prayer

Alex was getting ready to die. I could sense it, but I don't think Susie had realized it as yet. If she had, she wasn't letting herself believe it. There was nothing more that could be done but to make Alex as comfortable as possible. Late that night I expressed my belief to the resident on duty that the end was near. She asked me what we wanted to do if Alex stopped breathing. I said, "Nothing." She said, "You know, Mr. Graham, I can't do that without having something in writing. The next morning, they brought the paperwork required to transfer care to hospice, and the reality of it all seemed to take Susie by surprise. We signed the documents, and to all outward appearances nothing seemed out of the ordinary. Alex continued to have the same nurses and the same doctors, only now a pain-management specialist was also on duty. We didn't tell Alex that the specialist was from hospice.

A friend stopped by and I told him, "Alex is not going to be with us much longer." He asked, "Bill, what can I do?" He, like so many family and friends and strangers from the community, wanted to do whatever they could to help. The love and caring they showed over that past year was unbelievable. Most of the time they didn't know what to say, but they came anyway. They showed a lot of heart and a lot of courage.

For me, that's what it gets down to. The bottom line is courage. I believe that when we are faced with tragedy, especially an illness like cancer, our first instinct is avoidance. We don't want to deal with it, because in a way if we do, we are forced to face our own mortality. So, there are those who turn the other way, and there are those who overcome their uneasiness and choose to be there for you. They still may not know exactly what to say, but they summon the courage to do the right thing, and they come to your aid.

When my courageous friend asked what he could do, I didn't know quite how to answer. I finally said, "E-mail Ed." I knew Alex would want Ed Robertson to know. BNL was on tour in London, England, and I knew it was unlikely they would see the message anytime soon.

A couple of hours later, Alex died in the arms of her mother as I embraced them both.

Somehow Ed saw the e-mail and phoned us that afternoon. We talked for about 45 minutes. It was a difficult conversation, but I told him about everything that had happened. It was difficult, but at the same time it was comforting. It was comforting, because I knew Ed had been through tragedy as well. A few years earlier, he lost his older brother, Doug, in a motorcycle accident, and recently BNL's multi-instrumentalist, Kevin Hearn, was diagnosed and going through treatment for leukemia. Ed didn't have to ask the unanswerable question, "How was I holding up?" He didn't have to ask because he knew.

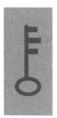

Courage is resistance to fear, mastery of fear—not absence of fear.

Mark Twain
American humanist, humorist, satirist, lecturer and writer

When One Door Closes

The Legacy

As I prepared for this heartbreaking moment, one thought kept occurring to me. It seems wrong—almost impossible to think of Alex in the past tense. When we hear of someone's serious illness, we often immediately start to detach ourselves emotionally—to treat them as if they were already gone. But Alex would have none of that.

WORDS SPOKEN BY ALEX'S RABBI AT HER FUNERAL

When One Door Closes

Go Out and Do a Good Deed

Friend Sarah

Walking into the funeral, the first thing that struck me was the sheer number of people. There were so many mourners that they were standing everywhere, because every seat was taken. In addition to family and friends, there were people from all parts of the community, from all walks of life, and of all religious beliefs. It seemed like everyone had heard her story and was there to pay their respects and honor her memory.

Those of us who were her close friends remembered different things and handled the circumstances differently. Two of the guys Alex and I hung out with were among the pallbearers. They took Alex's passing extremely hard, and both cried from start to finish. Later they said they were so swallowed up by their emotions that they remembered little about what was said. They didn't even remember driving out to the cemetery.

The same was true for shiva, the seven-day period of mourning that begins right after the funeral. My girlfriend said that shiva was the only time and place she found comfort. Alex's brother, Robbie, felt much different. He had to get out of the house. He couldn't sit around and deal with the traditional setting of people offering their condolences. To let off steam he actually took a couple of the guys out in Alex's Toyota 4Runner and went off-roading in a large, nearby field. By contrast, one of Alex's nurses was there, and she was uplifted by the gathering and felt a true sense of celebration of Alex's life. It just shows how differently each of us grieves. For some, it takes the form of custom and ritual and for others it may be something far less traditional.

One thing said at the funeral that made a lasting impression on me was the request made by the Grahams. They requested that for those of us who wished to truly honor Alex, it was best do so by performing a kind deed for another human being such as giving blood, feeding the hungry, visiting or calling a sick child or by making a contribution to the Beaumont Pediatric Hematology and Oncology Fund. As I reflect on that time and place and in talking to others who were there, I sense that request touched the hearts of everyone. We all came away from the funeral, and later from shiva at the Grahams' home, feeling a need and want to do something positive in Alex's memory. That's what she would have wanted, and that is how she lived her life.

Even when she was at her sickest, she still wanted to help others. In the hospital there were always little kids who didn't have anyone to play with, and there was Alex, in the playroom keeping them busy. She was even concerned about the nurses and made sure they took time for lunch and an occasional donut supplied by the Grahams. Alex was always looking to help other people, and that is definitely what I'm about in my work today.

I became a social worker for the Therapeutic Day School in the Chicago area. We serve kids with severe behavioral and emotional disorders—kids who couldn't make it in the public schools. Knowing Alex and how she tried to make the best of all situations inspires me to do the same with these kids. Many of them come from very poor families and broken homes. They don't often have consistent, happy, energetic people in their lives, and that's exactly what Alex was for me and for so many others. Yet, like everyone else, there are days I get up in the morning exhausted. I just don't want to go to work, but I have a special source of energy. In my apartment I keep a picture of Alex. I keep it in a place where I see it before I leave for work, and when I look at it I can't help but think of how she lived her life. For one more day, that memory gives me the energy I need to be the person and social worker those kids are counting on.

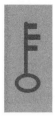

Death ends a life, not a relationship.

Morrie Schwartz
From *Tuesdays with Morrie* by Mitch Albom

Coming to Grips with Reality

Friend Jason

January 27, 1999

So understand if Susie and I don't appear to be the grieving parents. We've grieved for way over a year. We've seen Alex go through the pain, the discomfort. But the good news is that the pain of loneliness was something that Alex never knew. She was never in the hospital where she wasn't with friends or family.

Words spoken by Bill at Alex's funeral

As I helped carry her casket, the only thing I could think of was the conversation she and I had in the beginning. Her voice kept pounding in my head, "Am I going to die from this?" When she was first diagnosed we had the talk about dying, and I made her a promise. I promised her she would not die and that everything would be all right. We talked almost every day, and I always thought she would be fine. Now Alex was gone. I couldn't believe after all those promises she lost her life. After all we had in our friendship and after all the times we shared our feelings for each other, the last real conversation we had was an argument. The dirt was hitting her coffin and in my mind I was thinking, "I can't believe this is happening." I was in total shock.

That night, after the funeral, I drove back to Michigan State. On the way I got into an accident. I couldn't think about anything but Alex and all that had happened. For months I had dreams about her and conversations with her. It was frustrating that I had been so immature. Whether it was out of love or not, fighting with her was not the way we should have spent those final hours. Thoughts of her and our friendship would fill my head, and I would break down and cry. What a good person she was. She was such a caring and full-of-life person. She didn't deserve to suffer so much and lose her life. It was not at all like I thought it would turn out.

Some months went by. It seemed like I was starting to heal from losing Alex when word came that Julie, one of Alex's friends, had died. Alex and Julie met while they were both undergoing treatment at Beaumont, and Julie was one of the girls in Alex's PSA. She had been in remission for nine months, and everyone thought she had beaten her cancer. Suddenly Julie's death brought everything flooding back. Then, not too long after that, my mom came up to school for a visit and to take me out to dinner. That's when she told me that she had been diagnosed with breast cancer. My first thoughts were, "Oh, God! Am I now going to lose my mother to cancer too?"

My mom assured me, "No, son, I'm not going to die." She then went through the chemo and radiation, and she lost her hair. What was amazing was that through it all, my mother drew strength from Alex. She used Alex as motivation and inspiration. She said, "If Alex could go through all that she went through and did all the things that she did, then I can certainly make it through this." It was starting to register with me what a difference Alex was still making in people's lives, not only through her public-service announcement, but through her example.

Years later, I was going through a difficult period in my life. The good news was that my mom had made it through her battle with cancer, but not long after that, my parents divorced. Much had changed, and I was at a point in my life where I was upset about a lot of things and feeling overwhelmed. I felt sorry for myself, and I was frustrated about life in general. I sensed a sudden and urgent need to go to the cemetery and visit Alex's grave.

Once there, I knelt down and began speaking to Alex. I was talking aloud, and it was as though I could actually hear her voice responding. For me, at that moment, everything seemed to crystallize. How could I possibly go on feeling bad about anything going on in my life when Alex went through all that she did, accomplished all that she accomplished and now laid in the ground? Her life changed my life. Her death changed my life. Because she was strong, she remains a source of strength for me. She lost her battle with cancer, but she lives on in her message and in the hearts of those she inspires.

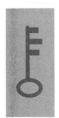

What you remember is part of you. Every memory I have is me...what a glorious feeling it is to know this! We each have the power to retrieve any piece of ourselves that we desire, and to experience it right here, right now in this present moment.

Wayne W. Dyer, Ph.D.
Author, *Inspiration: Your Ultimate Calling*

Death Is Not Dying

Ronald B. Irwin, M. D.

In her 17 years, Alex changed the world more than I ever will.

Alex's Orthopedic Oncologist

While on fellowship at the Mayo Clinic, I tried to do both general orthopedics and orthopedic oncology. Doing both is difficult for two reasons. In general orthopedics, the waiting room is always full and the practice is very lucrative. In orthopedic oncology, the number of patients is smaller. It is also the least lucrative of all fields because it is labor intensive with surgery and long recoveries. Insurance companies don't really know how to reimburse you for that kind of ongoing effort and involvement.

There is also a third reason doing both is difficult, and it is the one I find most compelling. It is a near overwhelming contrast to go from one room where you might inject someone for tennis elbow to the next where you are meeting a 12-year-old who may be dead from cancer in six months. A week later the orthopedic patient is 80 percent better but still whining about the discomfort while the oncology patient is going through chemotherapy and fighting for his or her life.

Orthopedic oncology sounds like a terrible job, but I find it the most rewarding. It is the best job in the world because of the relationships you build. Your patients appreciate you so much, because you are their last resort. I take care of people of all ages who have soft-tissue sarcoma, metastasis and cancers. That has been my concentration for almost 30 years. Of all the people I have taken care of, Alex is one of two patients I think of every day. I know that does not sound fair to all the others, but Alex was a remarkable individual. I will be forever impressed by the courage that she showed during her disease and her desire to help other people who were in the same situation. It was as if she was the counselor for the rest of us. She acted more like the nurse than one of the patients. She was trying to help other people deal with the realities of life-threatening disease, and that is exactly what she did with her unselfish wish. Her message and her public-service announcement changed lives then, and they continue to do so today. On a personal level, it was because of Alex and her wish that I became involved in Make-A-Wish and served on their board of directors.

It seems to me that many of the physicians and surgeons I know are not enjoying their careers. Often the conversations that I hear in the hospital, doctor's cafeteria and surgeons' changing room are centered on concerns such as medical malpractice, peer-review directive or inquiries or third-party inadequacies. In talking with other physicians, many say they would not advise their children to enter the medical profession. I am saddened by this and do not think it has to be that way. I wonder if we, as physicians, have lost sight of the goals we set at the beginning of our careers: that of helping the sick to regain their health, the lame to walk, to prevent death, and when that is not possible, to improve the quality of remaining life.

Physicians and surgeons need to put themselves in the shoes of our patients. We must be cognizant of their deep-seated fears about disease and their own mortality while realizing they trust us to help them with their problems. Patients need us to be expert in our various surgical and cognitive skills, but even more they need us to listen, to understand, and care about them as human beings. When I listen, understand and care, even if there is no cure, at least I am able to help my patients face their disease and our finiteness as humans.

Alex faced up to her situation. In fact, she was probably the most mature patient I've ever had, particularly at her young age. She took the disease and cut it off from herself. Through her actions she basically said, "Do what you need to do. I'll live my life. The disease has nothing to do with me." For a teenager, she had no trouble saying what she thought. She didn't have time for baloney. In addition to providing surgical skills and methods, I tried to look Alex and her family in the eye, to be totally honest, and to listen to what they were asking me about themselves and her illness.

I also try to let patients and their families know when it is time to make sure "their house is in order" both spiritually and financially. There is no way I could do this without a firm belief there is something better awaiting us after death and that we will all be with God when our sojourn on earth is over. Alex was Jewish, and I was brought up Christian. Both of us were strengthened by our individual faith, yet we shared a common bond. The reason that I wear this necklace with nine points is because the points represent the nine major religions that believe in one God. I believe we all worship the same God and that death is not dying. I believe that again one day I am going to see my patients who lost their lives to disease. I am going to see Alex and these kids with their legs and arms intact. That's what I believe.

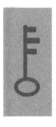

God is a resource. The energy of hope and faith is always available. We must all die someday, but the spiritual way is always open to everyone and can make our lives beautiful whenever we choose it.

Bernie S. Siegel, M.D.
Author, *Love, Medicine & Miracles*

Letting Go and Holding On

Friend Sharone

As a teenager, when your best friend dies, you not only lose your friend, you lose your own invincibility factor. I suddenly realized life can be over from anything at anytime.

Friend of Alex

There had never been a friend in my life that had faced a life-threatening illness. I associated cancer with people who were older. When my friend Alex was diagnosed I was petrified. I didn't understand it. I associated cancer with a death sentence. I was confused, and I was angry. As time went on, Alex fought hard and tried to live life to the fullest. I truly believed she was going to make it. In the end, when she was gone, I felt let down. She worked so hard, she had such a good attitude and she did everything right. Everyone worked so hard. How could this happen? I found myself angry again.

I could not tell you one thing that was said at the funeral. I remember looking around and seeing so many people there. Many had to stand because every seat was filled. I looked at her in the casket and kept thinking that she would open her eyes. I didn't want to stop looking, because I knew it would be the last time I would see her. She wasn't dead to me. She would never be dead to me. It was strange, because I was angrier about seeing her like that than I was sad. For some reason I didn't want to cry. I was angry and wanted to be left alone. I mean, what if she would have just had the amputation from the knee down right from the beginning instead of trying chemo? Why had she been so stubborn? Who cared about her running? I cared about her living, and in the end she wasn't able to run, anyway. Now she was gone.

It took time to let go of the intense, emotional anger I was feeling. As the years go by, I gain perspective on what happened and learn to focus on the good memories Alex and I shared. I have made a conscious effort to release the sadness, embrace the positive and appreciate the lessons learned.

My parents were responsible for one of those lessons. Had they prevented me from being there for Alex, it could have easily caused stress in our relationship. Looking back and thinking about how strict they typically were, I find the degree of freedom they allowed me was amazing. When it came to Alex, it was one area of my life where they said nothing to limit or discourage me. In fact, they encouraged me. For example, back then I was an inexperienced driver, and yet they let me take the car across town to spend as much time as I needed with Alex. They didn't ask a million questions or quiz me on when I would be home. They even let me take that trip to Memorial Sloan-Kettering in New York to be with Alex for her lung surgery. And, whenever I came home from being with Alex, they were sensitive to my moods. If I was upset, they would give me space. Somehow they could tell when I needed a hug or needed them to back off. That's the kind of parent I want to be.

Most of all I am thankful for my friendship with Alex and for how her wish changed my life. In college I was in a public relations class, and our assignment was to interview a PR practitioner. I was sitting in front of the TV wracking my brain for someone to interview and on came a message from the Make-A-Wish Foundation. At the bottom of the screen there was a name and the caption read, "Director of Public Relations." I'm like, "Of course!" I made a call and arranged to interview the director. Not long after, Make-A-Wish offered me an internship. The following year, in my final college public relations class my assignment was to create a press kit for an organization and then act as the press manager. I thought, "Well it was really because of Alex that I went with Make-A-Wish on my earlier assignment.

Good things came from that, so I think I'll stick with Alex and make a press kit for Memorial Sloan-Kettering Cancer Center in New York."

After interning with the public relations manager and the manager for corporate sponsorships at Make-A-Wish, working there became my dream job. I wanted a career with Make-A-Wish. I wanted to be the PR director, and that's all I wanted to do. As it turned out, there wasn't an immediate opportunity with Make-A-Wish, but I did end up working for a nonprofit. What's great is that I'm still able to work with Make-A-Wish as a wish-granting volunteer. I love the organization and their staff, and I love what they do for the kids and the families they serve. I'll never forget what they did for my friend Alex, and I'll never forget what her message did for me and for so many others.

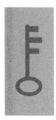

If you really miss and care about someone, take a little piece of what you thought was special about them and incorporate that into what you are today.

Source Unknown

What Would Alex Do?

Friend Paul

Alexandra "Alex" Graham
Beloved Daughter, Sister and Friend
May 6, 1981–January 25, 1999
"And a wind lifted me up."

The evening before the funeral, the Grahams invited many of Alex's friends to come to their home. There we sat in the basement going through hundreds of pictures. We cut them out and pasted them on two large poster boards to create these giant memory-packed collages. We talked about Alex and all the great times the photographs brought to mind. Making the collages was one of the most therapeutic experiences I've ever known.

Even now I carry a picture of Alex with me in my wallet. After she died I had it laminated, and it has outlasted four or five wallets so far. It is the only picture I carry with me. It's not that other people aren't loved dearly in my life. It's because carrying her picture is a reflection of how much Alex and her legacy still mean to me today. I can say this with certainty. Alex was the most important person ever to have entered my life. She is the person who has had the single greatest effect on how I act and the decisions I make.

Alex died when I was a freshman in college. Since then I have taken her memory with me and shared her story at every opportunity. I remember writing a paper about her for one of my English assignments. I ended up sharing it with the entire class and showing everyone her public-service announcement. Her story and her PSA turned out to be the highlight of the course.

For the remainder of the term, people all over campus were talking about her. And, on a personal level, whenever things got tough or I had a difficult choice to make, I'd ask myself, "What would Alex do?"

Applying to medical school was one of those times. Getting accepted was not an easy task. I had to take the medical school entrance exam twice and was rejected my first time. There were moments when I was totally prepared to throw in the towel. I thought about choosing a different career or getting a master's degree in whatever just to get something. But I couldn't forget that Alex knew of my dream to become a doctor and that she was my biggest supporter. I remember just beginning work on my undergraduate degree and, true to form, in the middle of her chemotherapy, Alex was getting me business cards from doctors and chiefs of staff. She was always talking about securing me an internship. Honest to God, when I thought of giving up on medical school I couldn't help but ask myself, "What would Alex do?" Deep down I knew the answer, and the only answer was to push forward, try harder, and not give up my dream.

I'm now starting my third year of medical school and am beginning to get some clinical exposure. What I have observed is a part of the medical profession that lacks human compassion. It's simply: Here's the diagnosis, here's the disease, here's the treatment. This is the name of the tumor, and here is how long you have to live. It's almost like a person's life is a frozen meal approaching an expiration date. But how Alex faced her illness, how she treated others and the message she left behind are constant reminders that there is a compassionate, respectful and uplifting role for each of us to fulfill. Those are lessons I intend to carry with me into my career as a practicing physician, knowing Alex will be cheering me on just like she did in 1999.

I still go to visit Alex at the cemetery and talk to her just like it was old times. I tell her about her parents, her friends and myself. I tell her the good and the bad, and I don't forget to share the humorous things, either. She would like that. For me the occasional visits are a peaceful cathartic. In keeping with Jewish tradition, I leave a stone on the tombstone, but not always one from the cemetery. Sometimes I bring one from a little waterfall in a local park that Alex and I often enjoyed together. Alex loved to visit parks, and she and I considered that particular one to be our special place. When I leave the stone on the monument, I smile, knowing that's what my friend Alex would do.

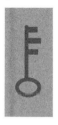

The most important single influence in the life of a person is another person...who is worthy of emulation.

Paul D. Shafer
American author

Try to Find the Good

Friend Amy

Have you ever met somebody
Someone special
They could turn your life around
Someone whose love is never-ending
Thoughts so insightful
In their feelings you could drown?
I've been captured by this presence
Don't want to lose it
I'm flying high above
And I've got to tell somebody
I want to yell it
I've been touched by an angel of love.

Excerpt from "Angel of Love" by Jeremy Wolfe
Inspired by a visit with Alex the day before her passing

A lot of people focus on trying to fix something that has gone wrong. Fixing things gone wrong is important, but my goal is prevention. Whether it's our personal health or the world we live in, the positive behaviors and actions we take now have the potential to improve our quality of life for generations to come. If you wait until a problem exists, there may be irreversible damage.

My degree from the University of Wisconsin is in zoology and environmental studies with a focus on freshwater ecology and toxins. After graduation, I applied to be a part of the first-ever human-powered expedition from the North Pole to the South Pole. The Pole to Pole Expedition will work with charitable organizations around the globe on the critical social, economic and environmental issues of our time. Through initiatives like Pole to Pole, I've got big plans to make a meaningful difference. I'm excited about my career and what can be accomplished, but I wasn't always that enthused about the future. If it weren't for Alex, my life could have gone in a much different direction.

I was 14 years old and feeling pretty much alone. I'm the first to admit that I was a bit different than most teenage girls. My background was more conservative, and my interests were less typical. It didn't feel like I had much in common with kids my age. Teenagers often judge you based on what someone says instead of learning to know you for who you really are. I had grown tired of all the B.S. and of trying to fit in. I had become more and more isolated. I was depressed and at a real low point in my life. Maybe that's not unusual for a teenager, but when you are going through it, it is very real and can be overwhelming. That's when I met Alex.

Maybe I should say Alex and I "re-met," because when I was seven and she was eight years old we had actually played on the same softball team. It was years later when I was in the eighth grade that we ran into each other again. I was attending a youth group event with my older brothers. Out of nowhere this girl came up to me and said, "Hey, I know you! We used to play softball together. Don't you remember?" It was Alex. Frankly, I didn't remember, but she did. Alex had a great memory, and later she even found a photo of our team to prove it. From that point on, my life and my attitude change dramatically.

Alex took me under her wing at a time when I was becoming more and more isolated. She introduced me to everyone she knew. She included me and made me feel like I belonged. Maybe I was a project for her. Who knows? All I know is that I went from a real low point in my life to being able to laugh again. She chose to see the good in me, and completely turned my world around. It was amazing to find someone in my own age group who didn't have a personal agenda and who genuinely cared about my happiness. Alex was a leader who used her influence to make me a part of things. She was confident in who she was and didn't need to exclude others to gain control or elevate her own status.

I ended up going to a different high school than Alex. Alex went to West Bloomfield and I went to North Farmington. There

I became very active in sports and extracurricular activities. That may not have happened if Alex hadn't "rescued" me from my unhappiness. Both Alex and I lessened our involvement with the youth organization we belonged to, and over time we began to see less and less of each other. That's when I got word of her illness. I couldn't believe it. My brother had just lost a close friend to cancer about a year earlier, so I had knew what could happen. I knew this was going to be a struggle. I knew cancer was a battle you could lose, regardless of who you were and how strong you might be. I felt an urgency to talk to Alex and spend time with her. I wanted to be there for her, because she had done so much for me.

Even while she was sick, Alex was still trying to help me out and make me smile. She was the one who was ill, yet she was the one showing interest and concern for me and others. She could have been consumed in self-pity, but she was the one asking, "So, how's your life?" Despite her courageous spirit and will to live, Alex lost her battle with cancer. I kept asking myself, "Why?" Could the cancer have been avoided? Where did it come from, and just how did it happen? Are there patterns that can be identified and causes in our environment such as toxins that can be linked? So it was Alex who really got me interested in prevention, and I draw inspiration from her example to this very day.

Alex was young, yet I think she had figured out the key to a fulfilling life. By example she shared it with everyone she met. Life is what you perceive it to be. You can become entrenched in the negative, or you can choose to see the positive. You can feel sorry for yourself when the trials of life block your way, or you can choose to live in the moment and take a new direction. You can be self-absorbed, or you can reach out to others. You can focus on the bad, the sad and the terrible, or you can try to find the good.

That's what Alex taught me. Just try to find the good.

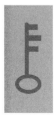

Just give love and unconditional acceptance to those you encounter, and notice what happens.

Wayne W. Dyer, Ph.D.
Author, *Real Magic: Creating Miracles in Everyday Life*

Handicapped Parking

Robbie

Alex was the kind of person who made decisions based on how it would affect other people. Her sensitivity to the needs of others left a lasting impression on us all.

Susie

Watching my sister go through what she did changed me forever. In the beginning, sitting in our kitchen and hearing my parents say, "Alex has cancer" was something I took in stride. It was an illness. She would get treatment, and she would get better. It was much different later on, walking the pediatric floor of Beaumont Hospital. Everywhere you looked there were bald five-year-olds running around holding IVs. There was this kind of weird look on everyone's face. It was as if they were hoping for the best but knew deep inside that many of the kids were not going to make it. That's when it started to set in for me. Yep, it's a lot different sitting in your own kitchen, talking about cancer while your sister looks the same to you as she always has. It's an "in your face" reality check sitting in a hospital room watching your little sister hooked up to IVs, skinny as hell, missing all her hair, and struggling to breathe.

The images of those days will never leave me. They are imbedded in my senses forever. Like when the hospital elevator door opened and the first thing to hit you was this unmistakable smell. Then to one side there was this waiting room. There were always boxes of Kleenex sitting everywhere, and some mothers and fathers were always in there crying. I'll never know how parents get through it. I don't know how my mother and father did, either. The emotional and physical load had to be tremendous. They wanted and needed to spend day after day and week after week with Alex. At the same time, they were still trying to keep their businesses going, and they still had to manage all of their other personal matters. Those days left lasting dark images, and I hate them.

But, even after all these years, I also have inspiring images of Alex that remain vivid and remarkable. The energy she showed while going through her ordeal was so amazing it was ridiculous. Who would believe that on New Year's Eve, just 25 days before she died, she was out partying with her friends? I mean, she lost her leg, and even though she had a prosthetic, she didn't like it. It was awkward, and it slowed her down. She would prefer just to have one crutch and go hobbling through her activities. To top it off, one thing that just blew me away was her refusal to park in handicapped parking. She was missing her leg, yet she felt she wasn't disabled. She insisted on leaving the spot for "someone who really needed it." Unbelievable!

That experience left me extremely sensitive to people who use handicapped parking and are not handicapped. One time, I was picking up my friend from the gym where he works out. The building was small and had about 20 parking spots. I noticed he left his car parked in a handicap spot. He comes running out and hops in my truck, and I'm like, "All right. You have to move your car before we go." He looks at me and says, "You have to be kidding." I say, "I'm not kidding at all. You need to move your car." He says, "I'm not moving my car. We won't be gone long." I'm like, "Okay, let me tell you about my sister." So I tell him the whole story about Alex, and by the time I'm done, he is sitting there crying. Hearing that story changed my friend, and I'm sure it's changed the thinking of every stranger I talk to when I catch them parking where they shouldn't.

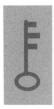

Those I have loved, though now beyond my life,
Having given form and quality to my life,
And they live on, unfailingly feeding
My heart and mind and imagination.

Excerpt from *Shall I Cry Out in Anger?*
By Rabbi Morris Adler

When One Door Closes

The Burden of Guilt

Friend Illana

When you are growing up, you have friends because you want to have lots of friends. This experience made me realize that I didn't need friends just to have friends. I needed people that would positively influence my life...people I could give something to and gain something from.

Alex's Friend

In the late summer of 1998, when I came back from summer camp, my friend Alex had made what appeared to be a pretty remarkable turnaround. She was on a special treatment of some kind. Whatever it was, it seemed to be working. She had color in her face, her hair was growing back and her weight was a little closer to normal. In fact, Alex's family planned a Northern Michigan trip to Traverse City and invited some of us to come along. We had a great time together, and I was feeling a bit less guilty about going to summer camp without Alex. I still have a picture of us together on that trip and will always be grateful to the Grahams for helping me and many of Alex's friends stay an ongoing part of her life.

Throughout her illness Alex was in and out of the hospital. In the early part of 1998, I hadn't been driving long and my parents hardly ever let me drive the car. They would, however, let me take it to Beaumont Hospital to see Alex. When I visited, much of the time she'd be sleeping. At the times she was up and feeling okay, she acted like a hostess trying to make sure I was comfortable. I'd be like, "Alex, I'm just fine." She'd scoot over on the bed, and I'd lay in the bed with her. We'd watch TV and read magazines and gossip. What we didn't talk about was what she was going through emotionally. She would complain a bit about where it hurt and the phantom pain and such, but for the most part we acted like any two teenage girls would act. Amazingly, she was the one concerned over the comfort of her visitors and wanting all of us to be happy.

In her final months, Alex became very skinny. To me she looked like a walking skeleton. Her back would hurt, and she would ask me to rub it for her. It got harder and harder for me to do, because she was so very thin. She seemed fragile. It felt like I was going to break her. It got to the point that I couldn't handle it. I wanted to rub her back to help her, but even though it sounds bad, I didn't want to touch her. It was too difficult for me, so when I didn't help, she began to show her frustration. Then, toward the end when she didn't even want to look at food, she would sometimes be upset when I encouraged her to eat. I always believed she was going to be all right, but when she wouldn't eat, I felt like it was the food that would save her. In my mind I was thinking not so much about the cancer, but that the lack of nutrition would be the one thing that could take her life.

I didn't really understand what was going on, and I didn't understand my own feelings. The whole situation was getting overwhelming, and I started to withdraw. I was a senior in high school. I wanted to enjoy that last year and have a boyfriend and do the things that seniors do. At the same time I fought a lot with my parents. They wanted me to pull back from Alex, because they worried that I was too involved. I'd get mad at them and say, "You don't understand! Alex is my friend!" I'd slam the door to make my point. I felt like my parents didn't want me to be friends with Alex anymore. I was drawn in different directions and didn't know what to do.

Then the call came from Billy at the hospital, and he told us, "You should be here." I arrived too late. Alex had died about 20 minutes before we arrived. I remember going to the phone and calling my dad. I remember sobbing and falling to the floor. When Alex died I felt tremendous guilt. I never regretted being involved, but what I did regret was pulling away those last few months. I was angry at my parents, too, for trying to pull me away. For years afterward I had these dreams of Alex. I'd dream that she wasn't dead but that she had been on a long trip. She came back and she was mad at me. In the dream she would tell me that we were no longer friends, and that she would always be mad at me. I know those dreams stemmed from the guilt I felt for not being there for her in those final months.

It took time and maturity to let go of the guilt. I haven't had one of those dreams for a while, and I am no longer mad at my parents. I know they were acting out of concern for me, and I'm sure they were only trying to prepare me for what was going to happen. I guess I blocked it out, because I didn't want to face the reality of it all. The experience has reinforced for me how important it is to be there for those you love. Just as important, you need to be there for yourself. I know too that you can't protect someone's feelings by isolating them from what's happening. There is not much that can be done to diminish the pain of losing someone dear, but you can choose to act in ways that will help avoid the heavy burden of guilt.

Today, I think about Alex with the fondest of memories. I think of her at times when something funny happens and I'll say, "Oh, I wish Alex were here because I know she would laugh." Sometimes I'll hear a song, I'll smile and say to my husband, "Alex and I used to bob our heads to this one!" And then I think about one other way in which Alex had a hand in changing my life forever.

One summer we had a chance to go either on a trip out West or travel with another group to Israel. I was leaning toward going West. Alex said, "Come on. Let's do Israel. It will be great!" I was persuaded, and on that trip I met a lot of new friends. Years later, when I was going into my senior year of college, I ran into one of the boys from that trip. I went up to him and said, "Do you remember me?" He had just started medical school at Michigan State, and shortly after that chance meeting, we began dating. So, I'll always be thankful that Alex talked me into the trip to Israel, because it was on that trip I first met my future husband.

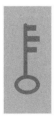

None of us can undo what we've done, or relive a life already recorded. … But if Professor Morris Schwartz taught me anything at all, it was this: there is no such thing as "too late" in life.

Mitch Albom
Author, *Tuesdays with Morrie*

The PSA

Jim Berline

February 5, 1999

Alexandra Graham's wish to raise the public's awareness about young cancer patients has become her wonderful legacy.

Excerpt from article by the late Bob Talbert, Columnist for the *Detroit Free Press* and Member, Michigan Journalism Hall of Fame

Alex's wish was to share her message with others. After her funeral we talked about that a lot. She wanted to get her "commercial" aired on television so that people who saw it might think differently of kids with cancer. She wanted them to give kids with cancer and those who looked different, a smile. She called it a commercial, but it really had taken the form of what is called a public-service announcement or PSA. Her idea of a home run might have been to have it shown a couple of times on the local Detroit stations, and I don't think she or anyone else had any idea of what was going to happen.

In my role as the chairman of Berline, I knew a lot of people in the television industry. We decided to make a whole bunch of copies of Alex's Wish, and I sent one along with a personal letter to the general manager of every TV station in the state of Michigan. In the letter I explained the story and asked them to run the PSA.

Before long I started to get calls from all over. It was airing in Grand Rapids. It was airing in Traverse City. There were people who had seen it locally on Detroit's WDIV. They had even seen it on CNN. It just took on a life of its own. When I sent it to WDIV, part of the Post-Newsweek group of television stations, it wasn't long before it was shared with affiliates in

Tampa, Hartford and Washington. Then I started getting calls from cable stations such as the one in Missouri who wanted us to send them a copy. Soon there were calls from everywhere from Vancouver to Europe. Alex's wish was truly coming true. Her message reached thousands of people, and I know it changed lives as sure as the experience changed me. The PSA even won the prestigious TELLY Award honoring the best in television commercials and programs.

You know, when someone makes the decision to start their own business, like I started Berline, everything is at stake. You have personal guarantees, second mortgages and you are trying to keep your kids in special schools. If you make one bad business decision, it can all be upside down. You become totally focused on making sure that you didn't make a mistake by walking away from a secure career to rolling the dice and chasing a dream. At the beginning, when we started to do some things for charity like an occasional brochure or annual report, it was done at a distance. Someone needs something so you say okay, here's the commodity you need. They say, "Thank you very much" and you say, "You're welcome. If you need anything else, let us know."

Alex's wish is the experience that changed everything for me. That defining event was soon followed by the loss of my mother and my daughter being diagnosed with a brain tumor. All of a sudden I had these three smacks of reality one right after the other. It was then I realized how easy it had been to get caught up in my own little world of making ads, chasing clients and feeling unhappy if the customer didn't love my agency's work. Those things have their place, but in the end, they are not as important as they seem. Instead it's the matters of family, friends and community that make life worth living. Alex's wish brought that truth home for me, and as a result I became personally and emotionally involved in making a difference. I call it being engaged.

I had the opportunity to serve on the board of the Make-A-Wish Foundation of Michigan for six years including two as the chairman. During those years we made sure we went to the hospitals to see the kids, like we do today with the children's charity CATCH. We go to Detroit Children's Hospital, and we go to Henry Ford Hospital. We see the things CATCH does to make a difference in these kids' lives. Selfishly, when you help out, you feel better about yourself, but you also know what you are doing is important and vital. You know that's true when you see the smiles on the children's faces. You realize it didn't take a whole lot of effort or time to make someone feel better.

I still use the PSA *Alex's Wish* in my business today. When we are presenting to a new client, we get them all hyped-up with a selection of our work samples. As an agency my employees and suppliers create some exceptional products. At the end of the presentation I share Alex's story and show them her video. After the client watches *Alex's Wish*, I sometimes have to make a special effort to lift their spirits before asking for their business. Yet it's worth it, because the PSA is a sample I feel compelled to show. Why? Because it speaks to the kind of company we are and indicates the kind of relationship we want with our clients. If the potential client sits there, looks at Alex's message and isn't affected, then I truly don't want them as clients. To me they're not real. If, on the other hand, they become engaged with Alex's message and show emotion, then they are more likely the kind of people with whom we want to do business.

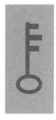

You can always find the time for the things that are important, and helping others is important. Because it's a priority, you find a way. Life goes by too quickly to wait.

Jim Berline
Chairman, BERLINE

Ed Robertson on Reaching Out

Ed Robertson, Singer, Musician and Songwriter, Barenaked Ladies

Just hours after Alex died, we got a call from Ed Robertson, who was on tour in London, England. He said, "Bill, Alex touched my life much more than I possibly could have touched hers."

Bill

The first time I met Alex was right before our CD *Stunt* came out. She was at an autograph signing we had in one of the Detroit suburbs. I didn't realize she had cancer. I just noticed that she had a leg missing. I thought maybe she lost it in a car accident or something. She was this beautiful, radiant girl and so excited to meet the Barenaked Ladies. I remember that she was just one of those people I felt a real connection with.

It wasn't until two months later in Los Angeles that I spotted her in a crowd as we were leaving the MTV Music Video Awards. I said, "Hey, I know you! I remember meeting you at that store in Detroit." She had made such an impression on me at that autograph session that even now in a sea of thousands of people, I went, "I know that girl!" I talked to her there, but it was in a later conversation with her parents I realized just how sick Alex really was. In the months that followed, she saw us perform in concert, and I had the opportunity to visit her when she was hospitalized.

That sort of thing is actually pretty easy for us to do. We try to do it as much as we can, but we don't do it as much as we should. When we do, it makes such an obvious impact on the both the people we visit and on ourselves. Alex made an impact on me. She was an incredibly positive person.

Early on in our career when we first started visiting hospitals, a doctor said to me, "These kids don't like to pretend everything's great. If you do, you won't connect with them. They're going through something that's difficult. Some of them might be in pain that particular day. So, what the kids will appreciate or what anyone involved would appreciate, is you actually talking to them." I think maybe Alex appreciated that. When I visited her I said, "How do you feel now? Does this treatment hurt?" I can remember talking to her about that and she would just be matter of fact about it. She said something like, "Yeah, it's not that bad now. It was painful before, though." So, I think when you try to actually connect with someone instead of just, "Oh, great to see you. Glad to see you're still hanging in there." Alex seemed really warm to talking to me about her cancer and what was going on with her, so I always felt comfortable and enjoyed talking to her.

When I visited her in the hospital, we actually talked more about her life than BNL music. I knew she was a huge fan, so I played the guitar and sang for her. She was a little bit embarrassed that it was all just for her. She wanted all the doctors and the nurses to come in and listen too. I said, "No, this show is just for you."

When you reach out and make those kinds of personal connections with a fan, it can be rewarding to those people, but it can also be rewarding to you. It's funny, we did another visit recently. We were on tour in Minneapolis, and we were really, really busy. We got a letter from a parent, and in the letter he sounded kind of angry and upset. The letter was about his 12-year-old son who was experiencing liver failure and had been through a series of disappointments with transplants. Understandably the parent was at wit's end. He and his wife were watching their kid suffer. The father wrote, "You are his favorite band. Could you just drop by the hospital?"

We were so busy at the time and we were thinking, "You know what? The kid probably doesn't even like BNL. It's

When One Door Closes

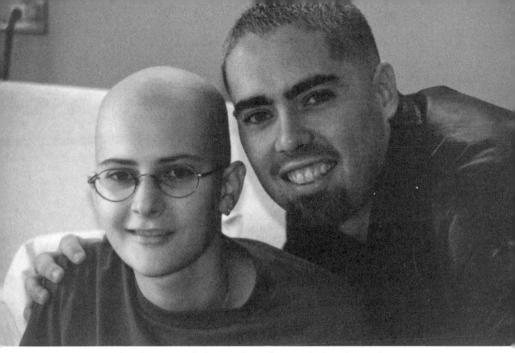

Ed Robertson and the members of Barenaked Ladies make time in their busy schedule to visit patients like Alex.

probably the parent who is caught up in their thing." Despite our preconceived notions, Steven Page and I decided to make the visit anyway. When we arrived, we discovered our assumptions were wrong. The kid turned out to be a massive fan of the band and a totally great kid. We came away from that experience going, "We just have to do this more often." Since then, we have visited more kids in more hospitals. We're just trying to make it part of our routine. It's not really that hard to do, and the rewards are tremendous.

Alex was one of those rewarding people to meet and know. I still think about her, especially when we visit the Detroit area. We have seen people with signs in the audience saying "Alex" or "For Alex." It always makes me think about how I would handle such a thing. You know, she handled it with such incredible dignity and poise. Even having lived so closely with Kevin, our keyboard player, as he went through leukemia, it baffles my mind how some people can handle it. I don't know if I could.

I felt we made a real connection with Alex. I know it brightened her day whenever I saw or contacted her, but it also brightened mine. I have great memories of seeing her, and I still have a copy of that video she wished for at my home, "We could use a smile." Now, that was a remarkable wish and a remarkable video, and I will always remember Alex as the remarkable, magnetic person she was.

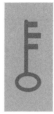

Life's most urgent question is: What are you doing for others?

Martin Luther King Jr.
Baptist minster and Civil-rights leader

Team Alex

Beth, Captain and Founder of Team Alex

I'm sorry for never having met Alex. I am most sad that she died and did not live a long and rich life. But, she is alive today because of Team Alex and your great passion and spirit.

A Team Alex Wish-A-Mile sponsor

I barely knew Alex. I just happened to be the mother of a boy who was in Alex's elementary and junior high school class. The most vivid memory I have about her has to do with something that happened back when my son and Alex were in the fourth or fifth grade. Some friends of ours had recently moved here from Israel. They enrolled their two children in the same school as Alex and my son. Changing schools for children that age is difficult. Moving to a new country and changing schools is even more difficult. My friends were telling us about the transition they and their children were making, and my friend said, "Some girl named Alex had called their daughter, welcomed her and tried to include her in what was going on." I remember thinking that was a pretty interesting gesture for a young girl. I didn't know Alex, but the memory of that act of kindness always stuck with me.

When Alex died, I took my son to the funeral. To be honest, I'm not sure I would have gone on my own. I mean, I knew of Alex and had met and been friendly with the Grahams. We were acquaintances, but we were not what I would call personal friends. I hadn't even seen the public-service announcement that Alex had wished for. At the funeral when Bill

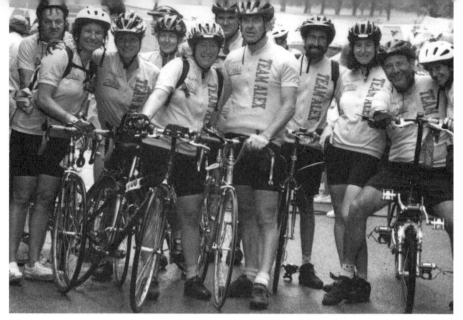
Team Alex prepares for another 300 mile Wish-A-Mile ride.

Graham spoke, I was moved by his message. Bill shared that Alex didn't want anybody to feel sorry for her. What she did want, Bill challenged us to do. He said, "Do good deeds in her name." Now, doing charitable works in the memory of others was a perspective I shared. What I didn't realize was that hearing Bill's message and taking a few simple actions would end up being a life-changing experience.

At the time, I had done a little bike riding. The longest ride I had ever completed was about 40 miles. I had heard that Make-A-Wish had a bike ride, so I thought, "Hey, I'll get a few of us together, and we'll ride in Alex's memory. We'll call it Team Alex. Maybe it will be comforting for the Grahams." We visited the Grahams' house during shiva—a seven day period of mourning. I asked them how they would feel about the idea of us riding in Alex's name, and they said it would be nice and appreciated. Then I called Make-A-Wish and found out that the bike ride called the Wish-A-Mile Tour or WAM was 100 miles a day for each of three days. Whoops! That was a lot longer ride than I had ever imagined, much less ridden. What was I going to do? What

When One Door Closes

would I tell the Grahams? Was I going to go back to them and say it's too far? And so, Team Alex was formed, and I became its captain.

1999 was the first year for Team Alex, and we experienced an incredible outpouring of support. Fourteen of us rode in Alex's name, and together we raised about $46,000. We didn't realize it at the time, but that amount represented about one-third of the total monies raised by the event. Word of the success of Team Alex spread quickly. It helped create awareness, and it raised the bar for all the teams participating. By 2007, Team Alex had grown to 60 riders, and it raised a total of $186,000 for the Make-A-Wish Foundation of Michigan. In total, the 2007 Michigan WAM event raised over $1,340,000.

Most of the members of Team Alex were acquainted in one way or another through our children's schools and activities. One of the couples who volunteered for the team had met Susie and Bill at the hospital. Alex was in the intensive-care unit right after her amputation, and their son happened to be in ICU at the same time being treated for a head injury. What is amazing to me is how through the Team Alex experience, my whole core group of friends changed. We trained together, rode the tour together and bonded around a common goal.

What is even more amazing is how my whole focus on what I do with my spare time has changed. When I say my focus has changed, I'm talking about a shift in how I choose to make a difference. Before, my efforts concentrated more on what I would call an "organizational charity track." That kind of work is certainly important and meaningful, but being part of Team Alex and WAM has brought me to a new appreciation for grass-roots, hands-on involvement. I mean, the idea here is certainly to raise a lot of money for Make-A-Wish, but that is only part of what happens. Large donations are always welcome, yet it's the hundreds of individual $10, $20 and $30 donations that reinforce a personal connection with Alex and her message.

Every year we send out letters asking for support. They usually read something like, "When you see a kid with cancer, or if someone looks a little different, don't forget to smile." We wear jerseys and T-shirts that say Team Alex. They carry Alex's message as well, and her message is underscored with a big smiley face. So, the story here is not about a group of people who went from riding 40 miles in a day to riding 300 miles in a weekend. It's about sharing the wish of one selfless teenage girl who had the vision to translate that wish into a positive, meaningful and forceful message. It's about the inspiration Alex gives us to ride beyond the aches and pains so that the wish of another child facing a life-threatening medical condition can come true. It's about the joy we feel when we cross the finish line to be greeted with a "Hero's Hurrah" from the very children whose wish Alex's message has helped come true.

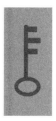

If one is lucky, a solitary fantasy can totally transform a million realities.

Maya Angelou
Author, *The Heart of a Woman*

This Is Not a Pity Party

Jason's Mother

Team Alex recently returned from a bike ride that raised funds for a crippled children's hospital. It was the most grueling ride we have ever been on. Of course, we could have all climbed aboard a bus and covered the same route in comfort, but it would have been meaningless. The bike ride had meaning because it was a struggle with a purpose. Life isn't all beer and skittles. We have battles to fight every day, and it's those struggles that give life meaning.

Bill

My son told me about a girl he met named Alex. That's not unusual for a teenager. Young boys are out meeting girls all the time, but he talked about Alex in a way that gave me the feeling she was someone special. I have these strong feelings sometimes, and I believe in fate and signs. This was one of those times. One day she came over to our house, and when I met her I was really impressed. Here's this pretty young girl with long brown hair. She was really adorable and had an outgoing, friendly personality. She was an engaging, easy-to-talk-to individual, not like your average teenager. I was thinking, "Oh, wow! If this turns out to be his girlfriend, that's cool with me." As time went on, my son talked a bit less about her so I figured maybe the friendship had cooled down.

When my son found out Alex had cancer he seemed devastated, and it seemed like he was talking to her all the time. What was interesting was that they had this fire-and-water relationship. They would fight. Then they would make up. They'd fight, and then they would make up. I remember saying, "Son, you can't get mad like that. She's going through a lot." I knew from the beginning things didn't look good, but my son was in total denial. He'd say, "No, she is my friend, and I'm going to treat her just like there's nothing wrong." When she would come over, whatever her condition at the time, my son would say, "Mom, treat her like there's nothing wrong. She's fine. She's getting better. She told me it's all going to be okay."

My son was a senior, and he and his classmates were on spring break when I heard his telephone ring. On came this young girl's voice leaving him a message. It was Alex. She was just beside herself, because she had just learned that they wanted to amputate her leg. She just poured her heart out to my son. Being a mother, I didn't know what to do. Do we erase it? Do we keep it? Do we tell him ourselves? What do we do? He's returning from his trip to a message that is so heartbreaking. We left the message as it was recorded, and that was the reality he had to deal with when he got home.

The amputation didn't stop Alex or her friends. They went to concerts. They went to the beach. It was amazing, and all along my son is telling me things like, "You know mom, they're making this special prosthesis for Alex. She's going to wear it and it's going to be great." At the same time, I would talk to my brother-in-law who is a radiologist. I told him that they took Alex's leg as high as they could possibly take it, and he kept telling me not to get our hopes up too high as it probably wouldn't stop the cancer. Even after she decided she didn't like the prosthesis, it didn't faze her. She went out in public without it and continued her life undaunted.

I have to tell you that the person I was back then could not have endured an illness like that. I also would not have been able to handle what Susie and Bill went through as parents. I could not imagine what they were all going through, yet Alex remained courageous and positive and her parents were unwavering in their support and encouragement. Her selfless wish touched us all, and when she died, the words Bill offered at the funeral are still burned into my memory. He said, "This is not a pity party. It's a celebration of her life."

Alex and her family changed my thinking and thank goodness it did. My son was just starting to get over the loss of Alex, when I was informed that I too had cancer. I wondered, "Oh, my God. He just went through this with his friend Alex. How am I ever going to tell him I have cancer?" That's when I thought, "What would Alex do?" I had to let him know what was happening, so somehow I mustered the courage to tell him. It was like Alex was now this thing inside me giving me strength. I had never been a strong person, and I swear, if I had not met Alex and witnessed all she went through, I probably would have killed myself.

At the time I was in my forties, and my son was in his twenties. I had just started the process of chemotherapy treatments, and one day we were all sitting in the family room. To me my life was a bit like someone waiting for the electric chair. I was waiting for my hair to fall out. I was sick and depressed and waiting for the worst. My son said, "Mom, look at Alex. She never got to go to her senior prom. She never got to get married. Look at all the things you have had the chance to do, and know that she will never have those opportunities. She walked all over without her hair and without a hat. You have to know there are people who love you and don't care if you have hair or not." What an impact Alex made on my son!

That's when I realized that Alex, her family and my son had an unbelievable impact on me, too. I remembered a rabbi once said to me, "If you really miss and care about someone, you take a little piece of what you thought was special about them, and incorporate that into who you are today." That's what I did with Alex. I took the courage and strength she showed and carried it with me. It got me through the rest of my treatments to remission without complaining, and to this day helps me tell her story to anyone who needs to be encouraged.

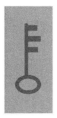

In spite of illness, in spite even of the arch-enemy sorrow, one can remain alive long past the usual date of disintegration if one is unafraid of change, insatiable in intellectual curiosity, interested in big things, and happy in small ways.

Edith Wharton
Author, *A Backward Glance*

Relay for Life

Jason's Mother, a Cancer Survivor

We discovered that doing things for other people gives a meaning to life at a time when it seems like you have lost everything.

Bill

The local staff of the American Cancer Society had heard about Alex and had seen her public-service announcement on TV. They contacted the Grahams to ask if their first Relay for Life in the immediate area could be held in Alex's memory. Susie contacted Alex's lead oncologist and asked him what he thought about the American Cancer Society. He heartily supports the organization, so Susie and Bill agreed to the ACS request.

I got a call from Susie Graham, and she asked if I'd be willing to participate. She gathered about 10 of us together, and I was asking basic questions like, "What is this Relay for Life? What exactly do you do?" With my busy schedule, I wasn't one to take on more than I could handle, but the enthusiasm of friends and family made it an easy decision. If there was something that Alex would want us to do, that we could do in Alex's honor while maybe helping another child, we were all for it.

Relay for Life is a community-based, team event lasting 24 hours. The event celebrates cancer survivorship, remembers those who lost their lives to cancer and helps raise money in support of American Cancer Society research and programs. The goal of each participating team is to have at least one member walking or running the course at all times. The event begins with an opening ceremony to celebrate survivorship. Hundreds of cancer survivors take the first lap around the track before others join in. For the entire event participants and visitors enjoy contests, prizes, food, music and a lot of good fun. At sunset, candles called luminaries are lit in memory of those lost to cancer, in honor of those who have beaten cancer and in support of those currently fighting cancer. It is everyone's favorite part of the Relay. It is best described as a peaceful and spiritual experience as thousands of candles illuminate the darkness and participants sustain their uninterrupted walk throughout the night. The event concludes at the end of the 24 hours with the announcement of how much the teams raised collectively.

The first year our Relay for Life was modest, with only seven teams participating. A windstorm moved through the area in the middle of the night, and lightning forced us to end the event early. Despite the obstacles we still raised $85,000! Every year in late fall when it's time to start planning for the next Relay, I always want to be on the luminary committee. That way I can make sure we always mention Alex during the ceremony. As the event grew, Susie and Bill have said, "Don't worry. It's not just about Alex." My friends and I are like, "Oh yeah we know, but for us it will always be about Alex."

There are now Relay for Life events in more than 4,800 communities nationwide. Teams of eight to 15 participants unite friends, family, businesses, hospitals, schools, churches and community organizations with the common goal of saving lives and eliminating cancer. Since my first Relay for Life in 1999, our local event has grown every year, and in one way or another, I know I will always be involved. In 2007, the Relay for Life that began with just seven teams has grown to more than 42 teams and over 1,500 participants. This past year alone our event raised over $363,000 to help open doors of hope and healing to thousands.

When I agreed to participate that first year, I did so in honor and in memory of Alex. Little did I know that eight years later as 4,000 candles were lit around the field, I would not only be honoring her memory, but I would be celebrating my own personal survival from cancer.

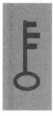

Take the first step in faith. You don't have to see the whole staircase, just take the first step.

Martin Luther King Jr.
Baptist minister and Civil-rights leader

I Walk for Alex

Friend and Cancer Survivor, Amanda

About four years after Alex's passing, we returned home from running errands to discover our house had been burglarized. I was speaking with the investigating police officer, and he asked, "Was your daughter Alex Graham?" He went on, "You have no idea. We have a child with a disability, and we were having such a hard time dealing with it. My mother saw Alex's commercial come on TV and she said, 'You have to see this.' We watched it, and I have to tell you, we gained so much strength from what she did and the message she shared."

Susie

I'm a cancer survivor. I walk for Alex in the Relay for Life.

It was February of 1998, and I was three and a half years old. I remember being really sick and being rushed to the hospital. On the way there I told dad I had a dream. I told him that in my dream I went to a really nice place, but he and mommy weren't there. When mom heard about it she said she didn't like that dream, and I couldn't go to that place.

When I got to the hospital, my blood platelet count was at two. They are supposed to be something like 200. That was the beginning of 28 months of treatment for acute lymphoblastic leukemia. Chemotherapy drugs are actually a poison. It's really a kind of experiment, because people all respond differently. You never know for sure how the chemotherapy is going to affect your body. There was even a time when I was taking 18 pills a day, and sometimes I fought taking them. I think I fought taking the pills because it was one of the few things I could actually control.

I'm glad it all happened to me when I was little, because now that I'm older I know more about cancer. Back then, I wanted to know what was going on, but it was never to the point where I was really concerned. I do remember that being in the hospital wasn't fun, and the days were boring, especially when I was neutropenic.

When you are neutropenic certain white blood cells called neutrophils are low. Those cells serve as your primary defense against infection. The low counts are a result of the chemotherapy. Extra precautions are taken to avoid food and plants that may carry bacteria, and there are often restrictions on visitors. When you are neutropenic it's easy to start feeling isolated and alone. That's when my friend Alex made time for me. She was a lot older than I was, but she would bring her Nintendo Game Boy, and we would play. Sometimes we would do art projects. Sometimes she would come to my room, sit on my bed, and we would just talk. We talked about what was going on.

I was excited when Alex asked me to be in her video. She wanted all of our friends from the hospital to be in it. When we went to the studio for the filming, we had lots of fun. They had a clown making balloons, and we got to have sandwiches for

Cancer survivors like Amanda walk a victory lap in celebration of winning their battle with cancer.

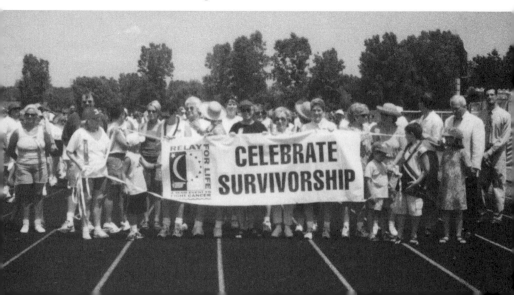

lunch. Now, when I look at the video, I can't believe it's me. I didn't have a single wisp of hair! I'm the one who says, "Too many pokes." Today, I'm in full remission. I've been getting good grades in school, and someday I'd like to be an engineer. This summer, I'm looking forward to going to back to Camp Catch-A-Rainbow. It's a camp offered by the American Cancer Society for kids between the ages of four and 15 who are in treatment for cancer or in remission. This year will mark my fifth year attending CCAR.

Yes, Alex was my friend. I remember the last time she came to visit me. She came to my hospital room. It turned out to be the day before she died. She sat on my bed, and we talked. I told my mom and dad about it. Mom said it couldn't have been Alex, because she or dad was always there with me. They didn't see Alex, and they knew she was very sick. Well, all I know is that I remember Alex visiting me. Maybe it was a dream…maybe not.

Alex was my friend. I walk for Alex in the Relay for Life.

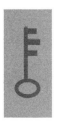

Some people come into our lives and quickly go.
Others stay a while, make footprints on our hearts and we are never, ever the same.

Anonymous

Stars' Guitars

Charles A. Main, M. D.

Our cantor would often come to the hospital in the evenings and visit Alex.
He would play his guitar and sing songs for her. When she died, we gave
him Alex's guitar signed by the Barenaked Ladies knowing he would use it
to bring comfort and joy to others.

Susie

I happened to be on the Beaumont Hospital floor
one day in mid-October, 1998, when one of my patients, Alex
Graham, was in for chemotherapy treatment. I approached the
check-in station at the entrance to the pediatric department and
standing there was a very properly dressed gentleman with a
guitar case in hand. He had already checked in and said he
wanted to see Alex Graham, so I showed him her room. The man
turned out to be Ed Robertson of the Barenaked Ladies. He
went in, sat down and sang to Alex. He spent a good hour with
her before packing up his guitar and heading off to his concert
engagement. Even before Ed's surprise visit, everyone knew Alex
was a BNL fan. Because of his incredible act of kindness, he won
over many more fans at the hospital who will never forget what
he did for one of their patients.

There is another Barenaked Ladies story that left a lasting
and meaningful memory for me. During Alex's illness, Make-A-
Wish was holding a gala fund-raising auction. Among the items
they were auctioning was a guitar signed by the Barenaked
Ladies. I was approached by someone who valued the positive
work of Make-A-Wish and knew the guitar would be something
Alex would cherish. He said, "I know you are going to the

auction and I'd like you to buy the BNL guitar for Alex Graham."
I said, "Okay. I can do that." He handed me a blank, signed check
made payable to Make-A-Wish and I asked, "What is my limit?"
The answer was, "There is no limit. Just get the guitar."

The only thing I could imagine that would be more fun
than going to an auction with somebody else's blank check would
perhaps be gambling with somebody else's money. At the auction
I remember feeling very relaxed. They finally got to the point
where they were starting to auction off some of the bigger items.
Among them was another guitar signed by a well-known
performer, and it went for something like $1,600. I leaned over to
my wife and said, "Boy, that's not bad." Shortly, the autographed
Barenaked Ladies guitar was up for bid. It soon became apparent
that there was someone in the far-right corner of the hall who
really wanted this guitar, too. I said, "$1,700," and there was a long
pause. Across the way I saw the other bidder talking to his wife
and others sitting at his table. At the last minute he said, "$1,800."
I countered, "$1,900." It was exceptionally fun, because I had free
reign. I didn't have to counsel with anybody. He would bid,
and I would go up $100. Back and forth it went until finally I
bought it for $3,400.

There happened to be other people from the hospital at the
auction and they said, "Doctor, we had no idea you were such a
BNL fan that you'd spend that kind of money on a guitar." I just
smiled and replied, "Well, all of us have our own little secrets. You
just never know." Later that evening my wife and I, still dressed
in our formal attire, dropped the guitar off at the Grahams. Alex
and a couple of her friends met us in front of her house, and
needless to say, she was ecstatic.

About seven years earlier we set up a college scholarship
program for our Beaumont Pediatric Cancer Center survivors.
We give each kid $2,000 a year, and we now have 33 cancer
survivors in college. Once they get the scholarship the first year,
they don't have to qualify again. If the college says they are a
student, they get the money. So if one of our kids was to go to
medical school, he or she could get the scholarship monies for
eight years. In fact, we just had one survivor who finished law

school, so she was given the scholarship for each of seven years.

Today our big fund-raising event for the scholarships is something we call Stars' Guitars. At the last event we auctioned 30 guitars autographed by different performers and groups, and the proceeds totaled over $130,000. I can't help but wonder how much of the guitar-auction idea was inspired by the night I bid on the Barenaked Ladies' guitar.

Alex touched us all with her courage and her unselfish wish. I still get goose bumps every time I hear "Wind Beneath My Wings" by Bette Midler, and every year when we auction guitars for survivor scholarships, I also think about Ed Robertson and Alex. I think about the compassion Ed showed by making time to visit Alex in the hospital, and I think about the smile an autographed BNL guitar brought to the face of a courageous young girl.

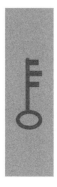

We survey patients treated from five to 30 years ago and ask them, "What message would you give to someone going through what you had to go through?" Their answers are the same theme: Take one day at a time. Don't keep thinking about way down the road. Just get through today and tomorrow.

Charles A. Main, M.D.
Chief, Division of Pediatric
Hematology-Oncology
William Beaumont Hospital

When One Door Closes

The Artificial Leg

Thomas M. Bremer, Prosthetist

When somebody loses a limb, the whole family is affected, not just the amputee. It's everybody. Life changes at that point.

Tom Bremer

The first time Alex and her family came into the prosthetics clinic for a consultation was May 8, 1998. Generally, an amputee wears a preparatory leg for about three months as her body goes through a lot of changes. There is always swelling and of course atrophy. It took about six different appointments before we finished Alex's preparatory leg. We tried to keep her prosthesis fit properly throughout that period, because a small change can make a big difference in a prosthetic leg. After that, we only had six months to work with her before she passed. There were times I saw her at the physical-therapy gym. She would put on the prosthetic and she would kick her hip forward and take steps. I was impressed at her determination and rapid progress. The first time she walked I remember exclaiming, "Wow! You've got it!"

I can only imagine what it would have been like to work with Alex long term. I know she would have done really well because of the spirit she showed and the strength she displayed while still in the middle of her crisis. She would have shown results in the top five percent. You develop long-term relationships with your patients, young and old. You see them a lot over many years as their weight and body changes. You bond because they see you as the one that helped them walk again and helped get them back into their life. In Alex's case, I only had the opportunity to know her for a short amount of time, but in that time, she already had an affect on me. The more you knew her, the more you wanted her around. You want to have caring, positive people like Alex around you all the time.

When a family donates a used prosthesis as did the Grahams, we are able to use the components like the foot and knee joint for someone who doesn't have insurance or can't afford it. People come to the clinic all the time who don't have the money or the necessary insurance. Costs can be as much as $25,000 or more. Ask yourself, "How do you ever go back to work or get insurance or anything without being able to walk?" So as a professional and fellow human being, what do you do? At our clinic, we've never turned anyone away. In the end, many of the people we help eventually find jobs and get their lives back. It only happens because someone cared enough to donate their prosthesis. After someone dies, even though the prosthesis is artificial, to the family it is still part of the person who is gone. That can make donating the prosthetic arm or leg emotionally difficult for the family, but when it gets passed on and makes a difference in someone else's life, it's a beautiful thing to see.

One day I got a call from someone at Northwestern University. One of the doctors there said they needed a prosthetist to join a volunteer medical group planning to work at a rehab clinic in Haiti called Healing Hands. Down there they had over 50 amputees with no resources, no components, no anything. They needed prosthetics, and they needed training for Haitians to run the clinic.

Haiti was a whole different world from what we are accustomed. We sent seven boxes of components, and the shipment was held up at Haitian customs. We ended up bribing them just to get our donated prosthetics into the country, and once there we found the conditions unbelievable. There were even armed guards outside our gates, but in the end the trip and the effort were well worth it. Today the clinic is up and running, and I've had the opportunity to return on several occasions. We have also had Haitian technicians visit here and work in our clinic. They stayed for a few months to learn more about their field, and then returned to Haiti with new knowledge and skill.

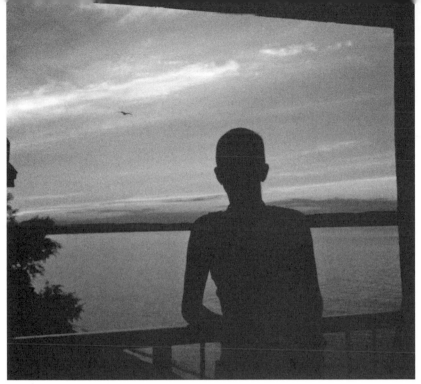

Alex makes a final trip to Traverse City, Michigan, one of her favorite destinations.

They are still working in the Healing Hands clinic, and it's likely that the components from Alex's artificial leg are still making a world of difference in someone else's life.

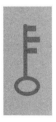

We have an infinite number of choices ahead, but a finite number of endings. They are destruction and death or love and healing. If we choose the path of love we save ourselves and our universe.

Bernie S. Siegel, M.D.
Author, Love, *Medicine & Miracles*

Like a Searchlight

Rabbi Danny Nevins

What happens if your prayers are not answered? If they are not answered, it is easy to think, "Maybe I did something bad." I didn't want to feel that way. I have a strong faith in God, but I've also come to believe there is randomness in life. That belief brings me comfort.

Susie

In 1994, I came to Adat Shalom Synagogue to serve as rabbi. That's where I met the Graham family. At the time, I was the youth rabbi and Alex was one of our teenagers. We were involved in youth programs and activities like our tenth grade trip to New York and mission trip to Israel. Alex was just this incredible free spirit, full of positive energy, not at all self-conscious, not differential. She wasn't cowered into respect and obedience by my rabbinic title. For me, we had a very natural, friendly relationship that was respectful, yet lighthearted and fun.

Initially, it didn't dawn on any of us just how severe Alex's illness was. She and her family remained so upbeat. When you would go to visit Alex in the hospital, you actually had to stop and realize, "Hey, I am going to visit a kid in a cancer ward." So, you tried to put on this brave face because you went intending to cheer her up. Instead, the very first thing she did was to cheer you up. You quickly found yourself drawing comfort from her as opposed to being the comforter. Actually, on a pastoral level, I think it was actually a little hard for me to feel like I was giving her something. Even the medical professionals who surrounded her, with their wealth of experience, felt as though they were learning from Alex.

There was something about her that wouldn't allow you to be phony or artificial. She had a piercing look which would search you out. It would silently demand to know, "Are you real?" You couldn't just say, "Oh, everything is going to be all right, Alex." That type of thing wouldn't fly. We had to level with her. She looked at you in a way that forced your mind to think, "Okay, I've really got to consider what I am going to say. I cannot just fill time with superficial comments."

When Alex looked at you, it was like a searchlight. It went over you and saw beyond the surface. In her PSA, there's a moment toward the end of the video when she turns her head from side to side. Her eyes cross the camera, and you have this sense she is illuminating your very thoughts. I associate that moment in the video with the image of a lighthouse as its light scans the sea. All of a sudden, there you are, caught in the beam for a moment. But unlike a searchlight, for those who had the privilege to know Alex, it was more than a temporary flash. It was a powerful and transformative experience. In part, Alex's tombstone reads, "A wind lifted me up..." The word "wind" in Hebrew is the same word used for soul. For many her soul is like a breeze, crossing through the land for a while but never gone.

That reminds me of something that happened just after Alex died. As a rabbi I get all kinds of unsolicited mail from many different organizations. Shortly after Alex's passing, I received a letter asking for used medical equipment to donate to patients in third-world countries. I called Billy and said, "I've got a letter that you might want to read. A group is looking for used medical equipment, and as I remember, Alex had a nice wheelchair. The letter is from an organization called Wheelchairs for the World."

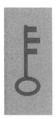

Why suffering? People have asked that question forever without much benefit. We don't know how God runs the world. What we do know is how to respond. We can respond to suffering by bringing a loving presence to those in need.

Rabbi Daniel S. Nevins
Dean, Rabbinical School of the Jewish Theological Seminary of America

Wheels of Love

Dorothy Pitsch

People ask me what was the trick in getting through it all. I tell them, "I took it one day at a time." I didn't have to go on forever putting on a happy face. I just had to do it that one day.

Bill

My husband and I had five children, and the two youngest were off to college. It was a time in my life when I was looking for something new and meaningful to do. I had prayed to God, "Show me some work that will make a difference in the world." That's when I got involved in a Christian outreach program called Wheels for the World. They gather used wheelchairs, repairing them and redistributing them to those in need around the world. They didn't have anyone in Michigan doing it, so I volunteered to see what I could do.

Well, I started a wheelchair-drive collection program, and they started to come in from all over the state. There were hundreds and hundreds of them, and it just kept growing. The wheelchairs continued to pour in. Somehow, the rabbi over at Adat Shalom heard about what I was doing and passed the information on to Bill Graham. Bill called and wanted us to come over and pick up Alex's wheelchair at his office.

It was a memorable morning. I had made arrangements to pick up a truckload of wheelchairs that morning and had an interview scheduled with The Detroit News. They wanted to get a picture of us loading the truck with wheelchairs to go along with the story. When that day started it seemed like everything that could go wrong would go wrong. It was raining, and the truck broke down on the way to our interview and photo shoot. The reporter just laughed and settled for a picture of us with some of the wheelchairs in a garage. With the interview ended, we were getting ready to go pick up the Grahams' wheelchair. As we were leaving, the reporter flagged us down. He had spotted our truck coming, so we went back and the photographer took shots of us loading the truck.

When we finished we headed over to Bill Graham's office to pick up Alex's wheelchair. At that point, I didn't know anything about Alex. I mean, we had picked up hundreds of wheelchairs, and this was one more to add to the effort. I walked into his reception area and met Bill. I recall he just looked so sad. He went into his office and came out rolling the wheelchair over to me. He handed me a couple of sheets of paper and said, "I want you to read these when you have some time." I said, "Okay," and thanked him for his donation. We loaded Alex's wheelchair on our truck and took it over to Surgard storage where we had hundreds of chairs piled up. On the way back home, I was reading the material that Bill Graham had given me. It was Alex's story as written by the well-respected journalist, Bob Talbert of the *Detroit Free Press*.

When I read the article I remembered my daughter talking to me about a local girl with cancer who recently died. At the time I had no idea who she was talking about, but now I realized it was Alex. When I tied it all together, I knew I had another very special wheelchair. I say another, because I also had one that had belonged to an 18-year-old boy named Larry from Clinton Township. He had passed away, and his parents wanted his $5,000 wheelchair to go to someone who really needed it and who didn't have the money or insurance to pay for it. I decided that I wanted Wheels for the World to track these two wheelchairs. I wanted to find out who got the wheelchairs and how the wheelchairs changed the recipients' lives. I called the headquarters in California and asked if it could be done. They said, "Well, we just don't have the manpower. You're on your own if you want to try." I was determined to make it happen.

I figured I better get back over to Shurgard Storage and get the two chairs I wanted to track. I had to find some way to identify them before our friends at Chrysler shipped them all down to Nashville, Tennessee. That's where inmates at a prison would clean them and make repairs before the chairs were shipped to their final destination.

Alex's chair was retrieved from storage and loaded in my car. I was driving down the road en route to my home when I heard this loud, clear voice. The voice urged, "Let's stop by and see my dad. It will make him feel better." I was alone in the car! Startled by what I heard, I sensed the hairs on my neck and arms stand on end. This was something I had never, ever experienced before. Then, while I should have made a right-hand turn to get to my residence, I instead found myself driving in the left-turn lane. I was thinking, "What's going on here?" Before I knew it, I had turned left and headed toward Bill Graham's office. I had no clue what I was going to say when I got there. I just prayed, "Okay, God, this is in your hands."

When I arrived at the office I explained to Bill's secretary that I was from Wheels for the World and wanted to see Bill Graham. She went to inform Bill, and a few minutes later she returned and said, "Bill thanks you and asked me to tell you that two ladies picked up Alex's wheelchair a couple of days ago." I said that I was one of those ladies and just needed a moment of his time.

Bill came out of his office, and I told him that I was thinking about tracking Alex's chair. I told him that I wanted to find out who got Alex's wheelchair and how it changed the recipient's life. I shared with him a story about one chair that was tracked. *LIFE* magazine published an article about how the chair went to an 11-year-old girl in China who was then able to go to school for the very first time.

Then with great apprehension I shared with Bill what had happened in my car. I told him about the young girl's voice that told me to stop by and see him and that it would make him feel better. Bill started to cry, and threw his arms around me. I was speechless. He then turned around, ran back to his office and shut the door. His secretary and one of his office workers witnessed what had happened. They came over to me and put their hands on my arm. All of us were in tears. I finally just nodded and walked out. I got back in the car and could feel Alex's presence. I reached over and put my hand on the cushion from her chair. It was sitting on the seat next to me. I whispered, "You're right, Alex. This will make your dad feel better."

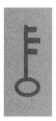

Whether you turn to the right or to the left, your ears will hear a voice behind you saying, 'This is the way; walk in it.'

Isaiah 30:21
The Holy Bible, New International Version

A Message from Maxwell

Dorothy Pitsch

Two semitrailers transported hundreds and hundreds of donated wheelchairs, walkers and crutches to a prison in Tennessee where inmates do repairs. One inmate volunteered to help with the restoration program and found his own life repaired in the process. He had been looking for a way to commit suicide until he started working on the "Wheels" project. He said it was the first time he had done something for someone else, and it gave him such a good feeling about himself that he felt like living again.

Excerpt from *Wheels of Love*
By Dorothy Pitsch

A few days after telling Bill about my plans to track Alex's wheelchair, I got a call from Wheels for the World headquarters. "We're thinking about you out here in California. How are you doing?" I said, "There's something I want to tell you. I need to share this with somebody." They got their photographer and reporter on the phone, and I filled them in on exactly what had happened. They prayed with me, and said they would send the photographer/reporter down to Nashville to help. He would personally take the chair with him on the plane to the planned destination, Ghana, West Africa.

The other chair I was tracking had belonged to a boy we called little Larry. His parents became involved in Wheels for the World and decided they would travel to Ghana and personally select who would get their son's wheelchair. They offered to help pick who would get Alex's chair as well. When they arrived they met a man named Maxwell. Maxwell was a leader for the disabled in Ghana. He worked with Larry's parents and the volunteer physical therapists from California. He showed them around, coordinated the distribution sites and served as an interpreter.

The villagers would be notified about the distribution sites. People with disabilities would get there any way they could. Some would be taken in wheelbarrows. The physical therapists would fit each person to a chair so that it would be the right size and meet their particular needs.

Maxwell himself struggled with the results of having polio as a child. While he was still a boy, someone had given him a small pink wheelchair that originally had belonged to a little girl. Now Maxwell was a grown man, yet he was still trying to get around in this little child's chair. After years of use, the wheelchair was in disrepair. The wheels would break off, and his friend would somehow wire them back on. Larry's parents noticed Maxwell's struggle and were impressed by all he was going through just to help the people from the neighboring villages.

The next morning, Maxwell took Larry's parents to the airport to meet the plane carrying Alex's wheelchair and the photographer/reporter from Wheels for the World. When Maxwell saw that wheelchair, he had this feeling it was for him. And thank God, that's exactly how it turned out. Larry's parents and the photographer gave Alex's chair to Maxwell. Maxwell, who was looking out for the disabled and others in need, received the chair from Alex. Alex, whose unselfish wish urged respect for the disabled and those going through treatment, forever changed the life of someone on the other side of the world.

Years later, the Grahams received the following.

Saturday, 12 November, 2005

Dear Dady Bill and Mama Sisie Graham

This is Maxwell your beloved brother and son greeting you from Ghana. Dady and Mamy how are you doing? I hope by the grace of God you are very well

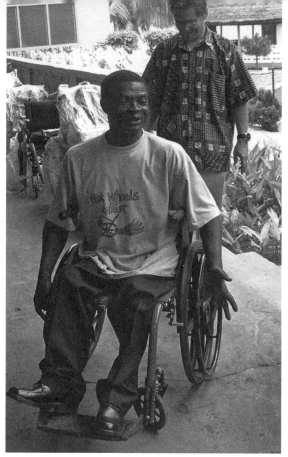

Maxwell enjoys Alex's wheelchair and his newfound freedom.

as we are responding to the same in Ghana.

Mrs. Joni was in Ghana for an outreach program and when I got her in Accra she has then finished distribution of the wheelchairs to Ghana. I am glad to tell you that I am still using Alex's wheelchair which was handed over to me in 1999.

It is now very old and I shall need its replacement. I have been changing the parts and I love to keep it so that I can always have the vision of Alex in my mind.

I love to hear from you. My family also love to hear

When One Door Closes

*from you. I am still on hot wheels for the Lord and
also reaching out to my brothers and sisters with
disabilities in my region.*

Best Regards,

Maxwell and Family

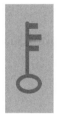

We walk the earth but once; we either leave a footprint or
go unnoticed...leaving nothing behind.

Dorothy Pitsch
Author, *Wheels of Love*

The Teacher

Friend Jason's Little Sister

One time I asked Alex, "Is this glass on the table half full or half empty?" She answered, "It depends on where it started." That's how we look at our time with her. We started at empty, but in her brief 17 years and even during the last 14 months of her life, our cup was filled with far more laughter than tears spilt.

Bill

I was a freshman in high school when I first heard about Alex through my brother and his buddy. I happened to be friends with the sister of my brother's friend. Being new to high school, she and I liked to eavesdrop on the older boys' conversations. They talked about these new girls they had met, and we thought, "New girls. Big deal." One time when we were listening in, they talked about some girl having cancer. It was the first time I had ever heard firsthand about a teenager having it. Since I had never met the girl they were referring to, it didn't affect me that much. I didn't even know what she looked like.

Then one day my brother picked me up from a tennis lesson. He had a girl with him in the car he introduced to me as his friend Alex. I had this feeling she was the one the boys had been talking about. Alex and my brother were joking around, and I could tell they felt comfortable hanging out with each other. I liked that she had this fun personality, and what I really liked was that Alex made the conversation all about me. She asked how I was and how my tennis lessons were going. When we arrived at our house she got out of the car, and I noticed she walked with a limp. That's when I knew for sure Alex was the girl with cancer.

After meeting her and knowing what she was like as a person, the seriousness of her illness became more real to me.

So I knew Alex, but I didn't see her all that much. When my brother was with her, I'd say "hi" or whatever. When things got worse and Alex had to have her leg amputated, I wondered if I should go see her. My brother was going to visit her at the hospital, and I think my parents were going too. I said, "Do you think I should go too?" My brother answered, "Yeah, she wants you to come. She said she would like to see you." I go, "Really?!" I had a part in a play at our community theater that evening, but there was time for me to go see Alex and still get to the play on time.

When we got to the hospital it was obvious she was in a lot of discomfort. Alex seemed out of it, but then she looked at me and asked, "So what show are you in? How is it going?" We talked about my show and the part I was playing. Our conversation was occasionally interrupted by her severe phantom pains. I couldn't believe in the middle of all this she was still interested in my little show. I remember going to the theater that night, and my own knee kept driving me crazy. I just kept thinking about it and about her and about all she was dealing with. I just couldn't imagine what it was like for Alex or her family.

I watched what Alex went through and saw firsthand how much my brother and his friends were hurting when their friend died. Later on, I watched my mother struggle with her own cancer, and I saw how she gained courage from Alex's example. After witnessing all of that, I too found that I could draw strength from Alex. Before I was the kind of person who would whine all the way to my doctor's appointment saying, "Oh, my God. I hate shots." I'd even be crying and feeling so sorry for myself. After Alex, all that changed for me. Now, in my head I go, "This is nothing…absolutely nothing." It's a life lesson she taught me, and one I will never forget. When things get difficult, I choose to think, "Don't be negative. It's not okay to think that way. Know that you are capable of overcoming obstacles, because if Alex could do what she did, you can do what you need to do."

A few years after Alex's death, I became a student at the University of Michigan. There I ran into so many people who got upset about the simplest of things like, "I can't get into the class I need. Now everything's going to be screwed up!" They would actually cry just because they couldn't get into the class they wanted. That's when I took the opportunity to tell them about Alex. I'd say, "Don't you understand? Let me explain what could be happening to you and how that compares to the thing you are upset about." Sometimes they would say, "Well, I have the right to be upset, too." I'd respond, "Yes, you do, but you also have to understand that you can choose to handle it in different ways. You can look at this as you didn't get the class you wanted and the day sucks and the world is over, or you can acknowledge you didn't get the class you wanted and find some other way to finish your graduation requirements." When something stops us from having what we want, we have choices to make. We can give up or we can choose to do something positive.

New York is where I now live and work. I'm a fourth-grade teacher and working on my master's degree. For my graduate school class I was given the assignment to create something that would be both meaningful to me and useful throughout my teaching career. I thought of my fourth graders. What really speaks to them and gets ideas across are true stories about people. I decided to write a book about Alex. In her own way she was also a teacher, and how she responded to the challenges in her life makes me want to share her story.

I call the book, *Alex's Wish* and it's written so kids can understand it. It describes her personality and tells how she was good in school and how she worked really hard. It talks about her friends and how many of them were kids she first met in kindergarten. It shows how Alex liked meeting new people, too. It makes the point that it doesn't necessarily matter what other people think of you, but it does matter how nice you are to others. Then the book tells about how she got a sore knee and how she found out about her bone cancer. It tells about having to have her leg amputated, but how even that didn't stop her from living life. It goes on to share the story about her trip to the amusement park, and how the experience made her choose a wish that was not for her own benefit but meant to help other people.

When the book was completed I read it to my students, and they responded extremely well. They thought Alex was really cool and tried to comprehend that she was only a teenager when she got cancer. They said things like, "My grandpa had cancer. My grandma has cancer." It was important for them to talk about those things, and it was good for them to think about the people in their lives facing a serious illness. It was also a chance for them to share their thoughts about people who had lost their hair or looked a bit different. What they really responded to was the part about Alex making a wish for others instead of asking for something like a trip to Disney World. After our discussion, the children and I watched Alex's video together.

I wrote the book because there is something for all of us to learn from Alex's example. There are core truths about the choices we make when adversity stands in our way. For me, Alex was a teacher, and now through telling her story, she can still teach in my classroom today.

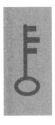

A teacher affects eternity; he can never tell where his influence stops.

Henry Adams
American author and historian

The Brothers Part II

Robbie and David

March 4, 2007

Radio personality Rob Gramm is shaving his head to raise money for childhood cancer. To learn more, go to foxspacelive.com.

After watching everything Alex went through and how she handled it all, it opened my eyes as to how precious life is. About a year after she died, I was out shopping for Hanukkah gifts and I remember thinking, "What am I going to get my sister?" That's when reality hit me right in the gut. I literally stopped in my tracks. It still didn't seem possible, but my sister was gone.

That's when I began thinking about the direction of my life. I asked myself, "Whoa, what am I doing? Where am I heading with all of this?" I was sleeping in all day and doing whatever all night. I had sold my landscape company and was heavy into the towing business. While it was fun at times, I wondered if a towing business was what I wanted to do for the rest of my life. I didn't think so, but I had no clue what to do next. Alex taught me to value each and every day, and her loss made me realize how quickly time and health can slip away. I knew I wanted to make some changes, but I didn't know exactly where to start.

One of my friends said, "You've just got to go back to school." I heard what he was saying, but I guess I still needed a sign from God or whatever. I just finished helping him move some of his stuff to his place at Michigan State. It was late, and I was tired, so I decided to stay for the night at his apartment. I woke up early the next morning and couldn't fall back asleep, so I got up and walked outside to get some fresh air. Standing there in the driveway, I spotted this guy at the house across the street putting up a "for lease" sign. The house was about a half block off main campus, and it was two days before the semester started. That's unheard of. Nothing is ever available that time of year. People are usually signing leases in the fall for the following year. I'm like, "I'll take that lease sign as my sign." I enrolled for classes at the university, and the rest is history.

I now work in the radio business. I began with a job at one of the local stations and one day sent a note to my boss asking, "To whom do I send my resume for a shot at the overnights?" Overnights are the live, late-night radio programs. One thing led to another, and before long I became known to the public as Rob Gramm, host of my own radio program. Today I am part of the popular drive-time show "Mojo in the Morning." I'm enjoying my work and living life to the fullest. That's how my sister Alex would live her life, so I'm confident she would approve and share in my happiness.

★ ★ ★ ★ ★

April 11, 2007

David's left kidney was removed early this afternoon in a three-hour surgery and it is now being transplanted in a 22-year-old recipient.

I was into carpentry since high school. In 2000 I got my builder's license and now own a remodeling business. I finish basements, bathrooms, kitchens and sometimes take on a small addition. Best of all, I am married to a wonderful woman, and my wife and I are celebrating the recent birth of our first child, a beautiful baby boy who we named after Alex.

Looking back, I have to say the experience that Alex and all of us went through changed me as a person and changed my thinking about life. It certainly made me look at cancer and suffering differently. Once you have actually seen what it does to people, how can you not help but change? It is one thing to hear about cancer. It's another to actually witness someone struggling to survive, especially if it is someone you love like we all loved Alex. Now when I hear of someone with cancer, I put myself in his shoes. I know what his family must be going through.

When my wife first started teaching in one of the local school districts, she met another teacher whose daughter had a rare genetic kidney disease. The girl was on constant medication and needed frequent dialysis. Without a new kidney, she was going to die. They were having trouble finding a donor who matched, so I thought I would offer to get my kidney tested. My feeling is that people shouldn't have to suffer, especially if there is a solution. In this case, because we were unrelated and of different races, who would have ever thought my kidney would be a match? As things turned out, it was not only a match, but it was as close a match as a sibling-to-sibling match.

The surgery to remove my kidney took about three hours, and the procedure to transplant it into the 22-year-old woman took about five hours. My dad said it was a joyful experience waiting with the young lady's family for the results of the surgery. The transplant went without a hitch. I'm pleased to report she is doing very well with her new kidney, and I am doing well with one.

Everyone told me, "David, Alex would be proud of you." I was always proud of my sister, and I bet she would be proud of me, too.

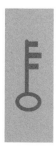

The recognition that the world is sacred is one of the most empowering of the many realizations that may occur to people with life-threatening illness and those close to them, their friends, family or even their health care professionals. It is one of the ways that such people heal the community around them. And should they die, it is often the legacy they leave behind.

Rachel Naomi Remen, M.D.
Author, *Kitchen Table Wisdom*

When You Have Been to the Depths

Rabbi Herbert A. Yoskowitz

Alex reminded us of how ordinary people can do extraordinary things when put to the test.

Alex's Aunt Miriam

When I was in the military service, I was among 40 chaplains chosen to receive special crisis-counseling training. Specifically, we were trained to help military personnel coming back from Vietnam who had suffered the loss of a limb. Our mission was to help them cope with the kind of physical change that is devastating to any human being, but especially to young, athletic men and women who suddenly find themselves deprived of arms and legs. They are in their condition through no fault of their own and are facing a difficult rehabilitation and an uphill emotional battle.

Why do I bring that up? I mention it because many years later as a rabbi of Adat Shalom, I was visiting one of our hospitalized members, Alex Graham. It was just after she had her cancerous right leg amputated in an effort to save her life. Her whole world had changed. I thought of the terrible trauma this young, athletic person faced losing her limb just like the military personnel who I counseled years earlier. She probably would never again play softball, run track, or enjoy the level of activity she once did. Then again, I saw something in Alex that I did not see in most of my earlier experiences.

The injured men I counseled years before were usually filled with extreme anger. The words they used to express their feelings were filled with strong epithets. If given the opportunity to reach for a drink to drown their sorrows, many of them would have. To have seen the same anger in Alex would not have surprised me, but what I saw was something very different. When I walked into her hospital room I found a young woman who was more reconciled to what had happened. She recognized what happened was not because of anything she did. It simply occurred. I was taken by the way she was able to focus on her person and not what was missing. I also noted how her family and friends didn't dwell on the absence of a leg, but on Alex the person.

I was there in the hours before Alex died. She had reached a point beyond the ability to fully struggle for life, yet by her demeanor she expressed her love for family. She was calm for those around her, and they were calm for her. My impression was that of being wrapped in a tallit—a prayer shawl. They covered each other with a shawl of comfort and peace. It's the image of the strong saying, "Here, let me protect you." Then the person with limited strength replying, "No, no, let me protect you." The challenge in life is for the ordinary to become extraordinary in the face of adversity, and that's exactly the challenge in life that Alex and her family faced. It's about how ordinary, in every good sense of the word, people can become extraordinary. Sometimes the situation allows it, and sometimes it even requires it. Some of us fail in that challenge. Some of us, like Alex, succeed. She rose to the heights.

Years later, in May of 2006, I faced a trauma of my own. In less than a two-day period, my whole world changed. I received a call on my cell phone and learned my mother had died. Ironically, I was already in my parents' hometown of Brooklyn, having flown there immediately after hearing my father was critically ill. While my brother and I were not able to be at my mom's side when she died, we sat with my dad, saying loving words to him as his body moved toward death. When he died, our status immediately changed. We became "orphans." At that moment I was not "the rabbi." I became what Susie Graham called "a member of a prestigious club I did not choose." Then, less than a day after my father's death, my only brother died of a heart attack.

I remembered that at each of my parents' 90th birthday celebrations they said their lives were complete. That gave me some comfort, but my brother's death was another matter. Like Alex, his song of life was not completely sung. He had so much living and giving to do.

My parents and my brother died within a 28-hour period. I wrote about them during shloshim, the 30 days of mourning, and found brilliance in the Jewish rituals of kriah, shiva, Kaddish and the Kaddish minyan. Yet, I really hadn't fully dealt with my loss. Grieving for my entire biological family was much harder than I ever could have anticipated.

One day, Bill Graham sent me a note saying, "Whenever you want, we can talk." A few months later we went out to lunch. I knew Bill had been to the depths of grief and felt he was one of the few people who could really help me, and he did. He said, "Sometimes it's just like a typhoon, these feelings that come over you and me. We have to ride out the wave."

At the time of my loss, people went out of their way to be with me. Because I'm a community person, hundreds of people came to give me comfort. I cherish many beautiful stories of their caring and support. I also remember one well-intentioned person who came to me and said, "Rabbi, how are you doing?" In my own mind I thought, "How does he think I am going to answer? Am I going to say "okay" or "I'm doing well?" How do you do "well" when you are grieving? By contrast, my discussion with Billy over lunch was among the most memorable, because I knew he too had been to the depths of grief. We are assured by the psalmist that although we walk through the valley of death, we come out on the other side. Psalm 23 reads, "Yea though I walk through the valley of death, I will fear no evil: thy rod and thy staff they comfort me."

You have to go through it. You can't go around it, but you

can reach the other side. Because of Alex, I knew Billy had gone through that door and traveled that path, and when we grieve, it's exactly like he said. We find ourselves in the middle of a typhoon, and somehow we have to ride out the wave.

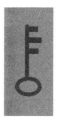

Trust God to enter into your pain and make it less painful, less frightening. Move on, taking one step and then another, no matter how dark the valley in which you find yourself.

Harold S. Kushner
Author, *The Lord Is My Shepherd: Healing Wisdom of the Twenty-Third Psalm*

With Gratitude and Joy

Cousin Karen, Cancer Survivor

What I find sad is that some people don't even look for new doors.
Alex not only found them, but searched for something good and positive
behind each one.

Alex's cousin

Maybe it was part of that midlife-crisis thing. I was
feeling a bit lost. My children were no longer living at home, and
I had devoted most of my life to my role as a wife and mother.
That was about the time my sister-in-law came home from
riding with Team Alex in the Wish-A-Mile bike ride. She was so
pumped talking about how wonderful it was making a difference
for the Make-A-Wish Foundation and riding in the name of
Alex. It was so inspiring listening to her that I said, "I want to
ride for Alex too. I'm going to ride with you next year." That was
in the summer of 2001.

Alex was my cousin by marriage. My children were about
the same ages as David, Robbie and Alex. In fact, my youngest
son and Alex were born only a couple of months apart. Our
families would get together for holidays and family events, and
the six kids would enjoy spending time with each other. We were
shocked when Alex was diagnosed with cancer, but even more so
when she died. She always acted so unaffected by her illness, and
we were all confident she would get well. At the very end, I chose
not to see her, because I wanted to remember her as the young,
energetic and positive person she was. I was devastated at her
passing. I ended up with big regrets, too, because I didn't get to

say "goodbye." I should have spent more time with her. Maybe it was selfish of me, but I did what I did. We all make choices we feel are best at the time, and have to live with those choices.

This time I wasn't going to have any regrets, but making the commitment to ride in WAM was a huge step for me. I had never exercised in my life. I did not ride a bike. I had never played sports, not even bowling. I mean, up until then I had a family to take care of. I didn't have time for all those other things. Now I had to start someplace, so I dug out this old, rickety Sears and Roebuck bicycle with a baby seat on the back and hit the road. I rode seven miles that day and thought, "Yes, I can do this!"

The first year I rode in the Make-A-Wish event was incredible. To feel the compassion of everybody involved in Team Alex, to see the people Alex had affected, to realize the thousands of dollars that had been raised totally amazed me. Through her courageous struggle and her wish, Alex had inspired them, and she and the participants in Wish-A-Mile inspired me. Because of their courage and commitment I told myself, "As long as God gives me the strength, I will ride this ride." Then, in April of 2007, my life changed forever.

I could feel something, but I didn't think it was a lump. It felt more like scar tissue from several biopsies I had over the years. I had always been religious about my mammograms, and this year was no different. I was right on schedule, and there had been nothing of concern for the last four years. There was really no reason to be worried. In fact, my husband and I were in the midst of planning our retirement, selling our house and moving to Montana. Imagine my surprise when on April 20 my doctor told me I had breast cancer. I had been riding to honor Alex's legacy. Now I was suddenly standing in her footprints. All I could think of was, "Not now. Not with everything that is going on in my life. I need to be healthy enough to ride for Alex in July. I don't have to ride all 300 miles, but I have to be there. I have to be in that community of love and compassion that Alex helped create."

The surgery was in June. Both breasts were removed including all the tissue they thought could possibly be bad. The protocol then called for chemotherapy followed by medication

When One Door Closes

for a five- year period. The minute I knew I had cancer, I knew a lot of things were going to happen, but the one thing I wasn't going to allow to change was riding for Team Alex. That was my focal point. I knew I had to work to get ready, so as soon as possible after the surgery I started walking. I still had drain tubes coming out of my chest, but I knew I had to keep moving. I had to keep exercising my legs if I were to have a chance at riding. At first my doctor thought riding my bike meant a couple of miles, but I finally got it through to her that it was much more than that. I usually trained distances of 20 to 30 miles. It was because of that training I went into my surgery very healthy, but to ride so soon after my mastectomy was a stretch. Everyone thought I was crazy.

Recovery from surgery was going reasonably well, except for a small part on one of the two incisions. Each incision was about six inches long, and both had healed except this one little piece on my left side. Weekly I would go to see the plastic surgeon for follow-up. She would measure the incision and see if the skin was taking. It was actually my skin attached to cadaver skin that was added underneath. Each time she would say, "It's not healing. Let's cut the dead skin off and stitch it back up one more time." I'd go back, and every time the skin would have died again. This happened three times and finally my doctor said, "You are going to need flap surgery." In that surgery they cut you in your back and pull through a muscle under your skin. They lay it over your breast area and take a skin graft from your back. The surgery is actually a bigger surgery than the original mastectomy.

I cried and cried, because my back is where I get much of my strength from for biking, and if I had that surgery I would not be able to ride. My doctor finally said, "Look, it's not healing, and you have to get on with your chemo. We have to get you healed up. We have no other choice. You need the surgery now." I said, "Fine, but not this week. I've got to ride in the Make-A-Wish event. When I get back from the bike ride, we'll do the flap surgery."

Two days later, I left for the Make-A-Mile 300. We started the ride on Friday, and I knew I needed to be careful. I'd been sick all year and couldn't train a whole lot. I never rode over 30 miles in a day, and normally in preparation for this event you would bike a couple of 70-to-80-mile rides. The first day of Wish-A-Mile I rode 42 miles. I thought, "Okay, I better take a break because I don't know what I am capable of." I rode in the van for 20 miles and said, "Well, I'll try the last 30 and see what happens." I rode 80 miles in total that day, and when I finished I hurt in all the right places. I hurt like heck, but in my legs and my butt, not my chest.

On day two I made my personal goal just to ride with a feeling of gratitude and joy. I wanted to ride all the way, but whatever distance I covered, I wanted to do every pedal with gratitude and joy knowing that when I got done, I was facing this real horrible surgery. Every time it was hurting me I just thought, "You think this hurts, wait until surgery next week." On I rode, thanking God that I could ride at all, thinking about Alex, remembering how hard her struggle was, and knowing she would have given anything to have been riding with us. I'd look down at my wristband, read Alex's name, and feel a surge of strength kick in.

I finished the second day after riding the full 101 miles. At the awards celebration that night, Billy surprised me by sharing my story with the crowd. Then he turned to me and said, "Karen, you are my hero." Suddenly 700 people knew my secret, and everyone rose to their feet and gave me a standing ovation. From that moment on, the rest of the ride was not the same. Every person, every volunteer, every parent, every Wish family, every rider who passed me along the way gave me a hug or said something encouraging. Whenever I took a break, they shook my hand and patted me on the back. It was so inspirational I rode the entire 93 miles on the final day, and when I finished the ride I felt euphoric.

A close friend met me at the end of the ride and said, "My God, I haven't seen you look this good in months!" I said, Well, I feel good. I feel tremendous." That was on a Sunday. On Monday I was so emotional over completing the ride and anticipating the surgery that I cried all day. The following Tuesday I went to see the doctor. She said, "So how was the bike ride?" I said, "It was great." She asked, "So how far did you ride?" I told her, "280 miles." When she heard the distance I pedaled, I thought she was going to pass out. You can imagine the look on her face.

It was time for her to examine my chest. She studied the incisions, paused for a moment, then looked at me and said, "I think you are healing!" I said, "What?" She poked me, and there was blood coming down. She said, "You don't get blood from dead skin. I'm amazed, but I think this is healing. Let's go back in the surgery room and sew it up again." The following week I went back for another examination, and it was totally healed. If I hadn't ridden for Alex, I probably would have had that surgery, and I may never have been able to ride again. Instead, I am on my way to recovery and riding for Alex again next year.

Some might say my blood supply was energized by riding or by the fresh air. Some may say it would have healed on its own anyway. They can say whatever they want, but as far as I am concerned, it was a miracle. The ride and the love shared inspired my body to heal. I believe miracles are out there if you are open to them, and my experience allowed a miracle to happen. To me, that is what riding for Alex and Make-A-Wish is all about. It's about making small miracles of joy happen for children and their families while they deal with the overwhelming burden of a life-threatening disease. That's a miracle we can all help make happen.

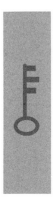

When we are weary and in need of strength, we remember them.
When we are lost and sick at heart, we remember them.
When we have joy we crave to share, we remember them.
When we have decisions that are difficult to make,
    we remember them.
When we have achievements that are based on them,
    we remember them.
As long as we live, they too will live;
for they are now part of us as we remember them.

Excerpt from "We Remember Them" by Rabbi Sylvan Kamens and Rabbi Jack Reimer

The Challenge

It's the Legacy that Counts

H. Thomas Saylor

The doors of everyday life come in all shapes and sizes. They can be inviting or foreboding, open or locked, easy to operate or impossible to budge. Open doors give us access to opportunities like friendship, education, careers, marriage and family, while closed doors test our faith, shake our confidence and discourage us from going on with life. Closed doors can deny us a job, end a relationship or break our heart. Doors can slam in our face in the form of financial ruin, an ailing loved one or an unfaithful spouse. They can block the path to our dreams when they reveal a life-threatening disease, a crippling disability or death of a child. Then, too, there are doors that deceive and entice. They bid us enter then tempt us to wander down roads of self-centered living and destructive behavior.

How we respond to the doors in our lives determines the type of life participants we are. Do the ways we face our challenges and opportunities reflect a sense of entitlement or a sense of gratitude and love? Phrases like, "Everything happens to me; I can never do that; it's not fair; my life is ruined; it's all your fault" are the slogans of defeat. Such expressions are the language of "victims." Someone else is to blame, and responsibility for personal happiness is relegated to chance and circumstance.

It's easy to feel victimized from time to time, but most of us choose to participate in life as "competitors." Competitors have their wins and losses. Competitors have moments of despair and negativity, but they somehow find a way to regroup and make a conscious choice to go on. They take on the new day and strive to make life better for themselves and those they love.

There is a third group of life participants. It's a prestigious group but one that extends an open invitation for all to join. In this group are life competitors who strive to learn, grow and teach. Its members are admired and emulated because they consistently make choices that open doors to positive destinations for themselves and others. These participants measure success based on values, principles and beliefs. Some live in obscurity, but many find themselves center stage because of the incredible strength and courage they summon when faced with the most challenging doors of all. We call these life participants our heroes.

All of us are participants, willing or unwilling, in life's reality challenge. Whether a victim, a competitor or a hero, we each leave behind a legacy. From the moment we draw our first breath until the day we die, we shape that legacy by the lives we lead and the choices we make. Tombstones have a dash between the date of an individual's birth and the date of their death. In the end, we leave behind the same little dash regardless of our years. That dash doesn't change because of how long we live, but it gains significance from how we live. It's not so much the doors we encounter, but the ways we respond to the doors—whether that dash, that legacy, is cherished and remembered or soon forgotten.

For heroes like Alexandra Graham, their legacy does not end with a memorial service or unveiling of a gravestone. It endures long after he or she has left this Earth. It lives on in the spirits and hearts of loved ones and continues to inspire. It is in Alex's living legacy we find and share a message of courage, faith, hope and love.

What Will Matter

by Michael Josephson

Ready or not, some day it will all come to an end.
There will be no more sunrises, no minutes, hours or days.
All the things you collected, whether treasured or forgotten,
    will pass to someone else.
Your wealth, fame and temporal power will shrivel to
    irrelevance.
It will not matter what you owned or what you were owed.
Your grudges, resentments, frustrations and jealousies
    will finally disappear.
So too, your hopes, ambitions, plans and to-do lists will expire.
The wins and losses that once seemed so important
    will fade away.
It won't matter where you came from or
what side of the tracks you lived on at the end.
It won't matter whether you were beautiful or brilliant.
Even your gender and skin color will be irrelevant.

So what will matter? How will the value of your days be measured?
What will matter is not what you bought but what you built,
not what you got but what you gave.

What will matter is not your success but your significance.
What will matter is not what you learned, but what you taught.
What will matter is every act of integrity, compassion,
    courage or sacrifice
that enriched, empowered or encouraged others to emulate
    your example.

What will matter is not your competence but your character.
What will matter is not how many people you knew,
but how many will feel a lasting loss when you're gone.
What will matter is not your memories but the memories of
those who loved you.
What will matter is how long you will be remembered, by
whom and for what.

Living a life that matters doesn't happen by accident.
It's not a matter of circumstance but of choice.
Choose to live a life that matters.

Courtesy Josephson Institute. See the Permission and Sources section of this book for permission details and information about the premier character education program, CHARACTER COUNTS!

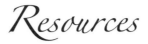

Resources

American Cancer Society

The American Cancer Society (ACS) provides educational materials and information on cancer, offers a variety of patient programs, and directs people to services in their community. To find your local office, call 800-ACS-2345 or visit the web site: http://www.cancer.org

When One Door Closes: A Teen's Inspiring Journey and Living Legacy

Please visit AlexsWish.com to find out more about this book, support materials, book signings, ordering information and special offers. At DoorWaysForYou.com you will find a list of available resources that can help open doors when you or someone you love is faced with a cancer diagnosis or other life-threatening illness.

Web sites: www.alexswish.com
www.doorwaysforyou.com

Make-A-Wish Foundation of America

3550 North Central Avenue, Suite 300
Phoenix, AZ 85012-2127
Toll-free: 800-722-WISH (800-722-9474)
Phone: 602-279-WISH (602-279-9474)
Fax: 602-279-0855
Web site: http://www.wish.org

The Make-A-Wish Foundation grants the wishes of children with life-threatening illnesses. The web site has information about their program and eligibility requirements.

continued on next page

Ronald McDonald House Charities (RMHC)
McDonald's Corporation
One Kroc Drive, Department 014
Oak Brook, IL 60523
Phone: 630-623-7048 (charity information and donations)
Fax: 630-623-7488
Web site: http://www.rmhc.org

RMHC provides information about local Ronald McDonald Houses on a national and international basis. The houses provide lodging for families of seriously ill children being treated away from home. The lodging is usually close to a hospital. The web site has a feature that locates a Ronald McDonald House in a specific area.